FACELIFT RECOVERY HANDBOOK

Disclaimer and Terms of Use: No information contained in this book should be considered as medical advice. Your reliance upon information and content obtained by you at or through this publication is solely at your own risk. Solace Massage and Mindfulness or the author assumes no liability or responsibility for damage or injury to you, other persons, or property arising from any use of any product, information, idea, or instruction contained in the content or services provided to you through this book. Reliance upon information contained in this material is solely at the reader's own risk. The author has no financial interest in and receives no compensation from manufacturers of products mentioned in this book.

The National Institutes of Health states that mind and body practices (now called psychological, physical, or combined psychological-physical approaches) are generally safe when taught by a qualified instructor. Just because a practice is safe for others, does not mean it is automatically safe for you. Do not use any of these practices to postpone seeking a health care provider (Mind and Body Practices, 2025).

ISBN: 979-8-9963352-0-6

<u>Important Notes:</u>

The tips discussed in this book were compiled through reviewing research studies and published literature and listening to clients. Experts may disagree and scientific advances may render some of this information outdated. The author assumes no responsibility for any outcome of applying the information in this book for self-care. If you have any safety related questions about the application of techniques discussed in this book, please consult your surgeon, primary care physician, or mental health provider. If you have any safety related questions about the application of techniques discussed in this book, please consult your surgeon, primary care physician, or mental health provider. Do not use any of the items or attempt any of the practices in this book without clearance from your surgeon.

Contents

Part One: Look as Good as You Feel 4

Why do People Get a Facelift? 5

Facelift Recovery Tips.. 8

The Facelift Recovery Rollercoaster 11

Tips for Reducing Swelling After Surgery 15

After You are Healed - MLD and Self-Massage............. 26

Part Two: Feel as Good as You Look 30

What's Making Us Feel Older? 31

Conclusion... 66

Resources 69

Part One

Look as Good as You Feel

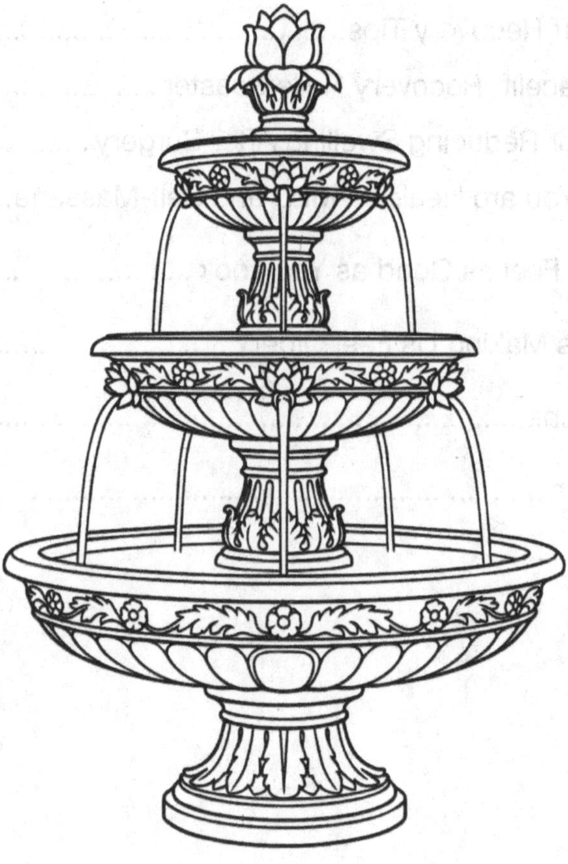

Why do People Get a Facelift?

Healing from a facelift is both a physical and emotional journey. I remember thinking to myself the night I had my facelift surgery, *Am I really this vain? Did I really spend all this money and now I'm feeling so sick all because I didn't like the way my face looked?*

As a lymphatic massage therapist, I have been helping clients recover after facelifts for over a decade. Having my own facial plastic surgery in 2021 has helped me to connect more deeply with my clients who are healing from facelift and necklift. I have experienced firsthand the fear, optimism, pain, doubt, frustration, embarrassment, and gratitude that come with the facelift journey. I can set their minds at ease that yes, the swelling does go down, the numbness goes away, and they will go back to looking and feeling like their best selves again.

Facelift and necklift surgery are used to treat signs of weight loss or aging in the lower face, jawline and neck. The surgery involves manipulating the superficial musculoaponeurotic system (SMAS). Most facelifts now also include facial fat grafting (Boyd & Ceradini, 2025). Many operations also include a necklift and blepharoplasty and some surgeons will also recommend a laser or peel treatment to improve skin texture.

Why does the face change over time? Some of us see these changes just due to gravity. For others, features like jowls or turkey necks may run in the family. Facial aging and fat loss can happen due to chronic elevation of cortisol and chronic stress. Changes can also happen as a result of weight gain and loss during multiple pregnancies.

Each person has a different story about why they chose to have facial rejuvenation surgery. For me, it was because the way I looked on the outside no longer matched how I felt on the inside. I feel that I'm still reaping the rewards over five years later. When I look in the mirror, a smiling face looks back at me.

Culture can also shape people's reasons for having a facelift. Research has found that people from different parts of the world have different reasons for undergoing facial plastic surgery. According to researchers, some people in the United States want to improve their quality of life, while some South Koreans are seeking personal and professional growth. People from both countries may use facelift surgery as a preventative measure. Some Saudi Arabians have facelifts for cosmetic reasons or to increase self-confidence (Rabah et al., 2025).

Having plastic surgery can change people's perception of your personality. Men who have had facial rejuvenation surgery are judged to be more likeable, trustworthy, attractive and masculine. Women who have had facial rejuvenation surgery are judged to be more likeable, have better social skills, and more attractive and feminine (Parsa et al., 2019) (Reilly et al., 2015).

Male patients who have a lack of jawline definition or too much tissue under the chin as well as men with heavy, thick necks have a high satisfaction rate after their necklift surgery. They appreciate improved jawline contour and increased visibility of the Adam's apple. Necklift may also be indicated to reduce excess skin after a previous submental liposuction (Bravo, 2022).

A rapidly increasing reason for facelifts is the weight loss associated with GLP-1 receptor agonist medications.

Researchers have found that over 8% of people surveyed who were using a GLP-1 receptor agonist medication reported experiencing a "hollowed out face." We may be seeing more of these operations, because the researchers also found that 11% of Americans have used GLP-1 drugs for weight loss, including about one-fifth of women aged fifty to sixty-four (Bozick et al., 2025).

Menopause-related changes may also be reasons for getting a facelift. Nearly half of all people having plastic surgery are middle-aged women, and many plastic surgery procedures, including facelifts, address the side effects of menopause (Malphrus et al., 2024).

Facelift Recovery Tips

What might be on your facelift recovery shopping list? Not all of these items are appropriate for every facelift. Please do not begin using any of these items until cleared by your surgeon.

- Baby shampoo
- Baby or child's toothbrush
- Button down shirt or blouse with a wide neck opening
- Cool-mist humidifier/essential oil diffuser
- Cold packs (not ice packs)
- Eye drops
- Eye massage roller tool
- Facial massage silicone cups
- Hair dye root touchup powder
- Incentive spirometer
- Jaw massage roller tool
- Mouth tape/sleep strips
- Powdered dietary fiber
- Quartz face massage roller
- Scar tape or cream
- Silk eye mask for sleep
- Sonic/electric toothbrush
- Tape for bruising
- Vibrating face massager
- Wedge Pillow (if your surgeon recommends)
- Wide toothed comb
- Xylitol products (if your surgeon recommends)

REMEMBER: Ask your surgeon before using these items and don't use anything not cleared by your surgeon!

A wide toothed comb and baby shampoo may be less painful to use if you have scars on your scalp. A smaller toothbrush may be more comfortable if you have trouble opening your mouth after surgery (Sasada & Guest, 2016) and an electric toothbrush provides vibration to your cheeks.

I used a wedge pillow to elevate my head after surgery, but not all surgeons recommend elevation. Check with your surgeon.

If you had an eye lift and find it difficult to completely close your eyes after surgery, ask your doctor if it's safe to wear a silk sleep eye mask to bed. This tip really helped several of my clients and improved their sleep. Your surgeon may also recommend eye drops.

You may find it tiring to chew food after a facelift. I enjoyed homemade vegetable soups, smoothies, diced fresh fruit and peeled and segmented mandarin oranges.

Your skin will be numb for a while after a facelift, so I recommend staying away from heating pads and curling irons as well as the extended use of ice packs until after you're fully healed. I used a small cold pack that I kept in the refrigerator, not the freezer.

You may have dry mouth after neck lift or rhinoplasty. Your surgeon may recommend using products with xylitol. Xylitol is a sugar alcohol and it reduces levels of Streptococcus mutans bacteria in the mouth. Chewing xylitol gum can also stimulate saliva (Yeruva et al., 2026). Tell your doctor if you are at increased risk for blood clots (Witkowski et al., 2024) and be aware that Xylitol is toxic for dogs. Some surgeons restrict alcohol and mouth watering foods in the first two weeks after a necklift. Ask your surgeon if you should eat a 'salivary rest diet' of soft, moist foods that are easy to swallow and avoid citrus, hard candy and gum as well as dry, sour, spicy, or salty foods if you had your submandibular glands trimmed during your necklift surgery. Be sure to read the labels on any packaged food or protein powder, as some of them can contain high levels of salt.

I used a humidifier to reduce the dryness of the air inside my home. If you have a water-based essential oil diffuser, it can serve as a humidifier, too! Another tip is to try mouth tape/ sleep strips when sleeping to encourage nasal breathing.

RED FLAGS: Call Your Surgeon Immediately!

If you are experiencing rapidly increasing swelling, severe one-sided pain, expanding bruising, shortness of breath, fever, drainage, vision changes, calf pain, uncontrolled blood pressure or sudden facial weakness, contact your plastic surgeon immediately.

The Facelift Recovery Rollercoaster

Let's first explore some thoughts you might have during the recovery process, then we'll look at tips on recovering from facelift surgery.

Facelift Recovery is an Emotional Rollercoaster

Crazy feelings are normal! Here are some thoughts I had during my facelift recovery:

The week before surgery - Should I really be doing this?

The first week after surgery - This was a huge mistake and why am I so vain?

The first month - What was the point of this? I'm an emotional wreck and I don't like my results.

The third month - Everyone else sees results but I'm still worried.

Six months after surgery - Wow, strangers are treating me differently.

The week before my facelift, I felt anxiety and stress. Did I make the right decision? Should I go through with the operation? These feelings are normal. Stress reduction practices are important during this week because severe anxiety before a procedure is linked to nausea, pain, and impaired wound healing after surgery (Wang et al., 2022). One source of anxiety is fear of getting a blood clot. Blood clots are a leading preventable cause of death after surgery. Calculate your Caprini Risk Score at https://caprinirisksccore.org/ and share your result with your surgeon. I will be sharing other stress reduction practices throughout the book.

During the first week after your procedure, you may be feeling disbelief and regret. For many of my clients, facelift and necklift is their first major surgery. We willingly paid tens of thousands of dollars and allowed someone to cut our face. I remember thinking, *Am I really this vain?* You may be worried about the scarring, especially if it looks like the scars are visible around your hairline. You may have bruises, and you may feel your stitches. You may be afraid if you move your neck you will 'break' something. You may feel swelling around the eyes, cheeks and upper cheeks, side of the face, above your upper lip, at the angle of the jaw, behind the ears and under the chin. Some swelling may feel hard, rubbery, numb, or like it's not your body at all.

You may have a dry mouth, and it may feel difficult to move your mouth and to chew. It may be difficult to close your eyes. You may not be sleeping well. You may be constipated and feel bloated. I experienced an annoying, low level of discomfort that made me testy. I wasn't able to focus on and enjoy watching TV or doing any of my hobbies. I was able to take short walks, but could not return to exercise. It's important to rest, because keeping systolic blood pressure under 120 mm hg can reduce risk of hematomas (Boyd & Ceradini, 2025).

At two weeks, many surgeons may say facelift clients are ready to return to work. Some people are, and some people aren't. You may still be experiencing all the things I mentioned from last week. You should NOT expect to look or feel back to a hundred percent yet. You may still be taking naps in the afternoon and feeling tired. You may feel lonely because of limited contact with friends and loved ones. If you are used to exercise, the lack of movement may be making you feel antsy or crabby. Your back and neck may begin to hurt from sleeping on your back. There may be odd patches of swelling on your face and neck and one side may be more swollen than the other. The swelling may look and feel worse than last week. This is NOT your new normal. You are still recovering from surgery.

About three weeks to a month after surgery, you might be experiencing feelings of frustration and disappointment. These feelings are normal and may be because the majority of your recovery is over, but swelling is still in the way of you seeing your final result. You may feel healthy and be able to return to work and activities of daily living but not yet look as good as you feel. You may still have bruising and your ears may still look swollen and feel sore or tender. You may be worried about when your hair is going to regrow around the scars on your hairline. Men may see different hair patterns around the ear due to skin being removed. You may feel zaps or a pins and needles sensation in your head and neck.

For most people, at three months, friends have noticed positive changes in their face and neck. If you're healing well with no complications, other people may think that you should be thrilled with your results. Sometimes we can get nitpicky and critical of our results. I have to remind clients that the swelling around the ears, jaw, and under the chin is still present. Swelling and induration may last for three months after neck lift (Morel et al, 2025). Scars will still be red. There may still be feelings of numbness and tightness. These symptoms take time to fully resolve. This point in healing can feel a little lonely. We may feel like there's nobody to share our concerns with, because the folks at our surgeon's office say we're doing great and our friends say we look fantastic.

Starting at about six months after surgery, I noticed that strangers began treating me differently. I think this may be due to a combination of looking younger, less tired and feeling more confident inside and that confidence changing how I took up space in public. I was carded twice for buying alcohol! This may make you happy or may make you feel frustrated as you realize how differently people are treated based on their perceived age and attractiveness.

Some clients have shared that some of their friends and family treat them differently as well. The decision to have a facelift is a personal one, and experiencing someone close to them having a successful operation may bring up feelings of envy, jealousy, and anger in those who don't believe plastic surgery is an option for themselves. For some clients, the people they thought they could depend on didn't end up being reliable, while people they didn't consider close friends did show up and provide support.

Dealing with stress in your life can slow down your healing. The client who is experiencing difficulties in their family; stress in the workplace; selling, buying, or renovating a home; caring for an older adult or caring for family members with special needs; or dealing with other types of chronic stress may have a slower healing time. Clients who don't have friends helping them or refuse help from others also experience chronic stress, even if they think they have "everything under control."

Tips for Reducing Swelling After Surgery

After my facelift, I felt terribly swollen. Dealing with swelling was the worst part of recovering from my facial surgeries. It was a constant reminder of the surgery. It was slightly harder to open my mouth, and chewing felt like a chore. Swelling made my neck feel tight, and the pressure felt like there was a strap fastened under my chin. Many clients tell me they feel embarrassed to go out in public after their facelift due to the way bruising and swelling has changed their face.

Our body uses the lymphatic system to remove swelling from our face and neck after surgery. The lymphatic system is our body's recycling system. It's a network of vessels that transport water, fat molecules, proteins, and waste products from the interstitial fluid in between our cells back to the venous system and eventually to our kidneys and bladder before we urinate out the excess fluid.

The lymphatic system is an important player in the healing process because "lymphatic vessels are critical for clearing fluid and inflammatory cells from inflamed tissues" (Schwartz et al., 2019).

There are several ways to reduce swelling, including:

- Breathwork
- Manual Lymphatic Drainage (MLD) massage
- Stress Reduction
- Vibration

I used all of these techniques in my recovery. REMEMBER: Ask your surgeon before using these techniques and don't try anything until cleared by your surgeon!

The evening of my surgery and the next day, I practiced breathing with an incentive spirometer to help reduce the risk of lung infection. I was really loopy on the pain medications and found it easy to sleep. If getting to sleep did feel difficult, I could have listened to a yoga nidra video to help me rest. I'll share more information on the benefits of yoga nidra later in the book.

A couple days after my surgery, I continued breathwork and added gentle massage. I began to help my lymphatic system reduce my facial swelling by gently stretching the skin on my neck with the tips of my fingers. Only a light touch is needed, because "the lymphatics of the anterior neck lie above the platysma muscle" (Jung et al., 2024). I placed my fingertips right above my clavicles and gently pulled the skin on my neck in a downward direction. I also used my vibrating toothbrush to brush my teeth. It kept my mouth clean and also vibrated the insides of my cheeks as I used it.

In between week one and two after my surgery, I started receiving professional manual lymphatic drainage massages. I also performed manual lymphatic drainage on myself in the morning, I could have also used a handheld quartz face roller or face massager in between professional massages.

Later on in my recovery, I started using a handheld vibrating face massager when I woke up in the morning to help reduce swelling. I kept it right at my bedside because my neck felt tightest first thing in the morning.

Let's take a deeper look at each of these ways to help our lymphatic system after surgery.

Breathwork

There are few different types of gentle breathwork that you can try after plastic surgery. Always get your surgeon's permission before trying something new. Let's look at three: incentive spirometer, diaphragmatic breathing, and cyclic sighing.

Incentive Spirometer

I was given an incentive spirometer to use after my facelift surgery. An incentive spirometer is a device that uses visual feedback (mine had a plastic ball) to encourage deep inhalation. It's used after surgery to improve lung expansion and ventilation (Kloni et al., 2026).

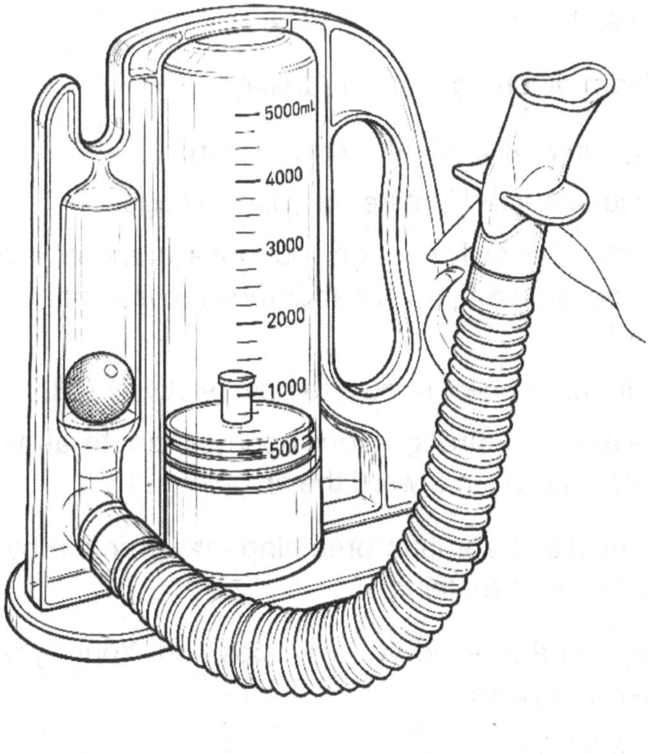

Deep Abdominal Diaphragmatic Breathing

Lung health is important after plastic surgery, especially after procedures involving general anesthesia. Deep breathing increases transpulmonary pressure, improving lung capacity, ventilation, and oxygenation. Slow belly breathing using the diaphragm also helps move lymphatic fluid through the deep lymphatics in our torso.

The diaphragm is a dome-shaped muscle located at the base of the lungs. Using the diaphragm while breathing can enable lymphatic drainage in the body. When we inhale and exhale, pressure changes in the torso move lymphatic fluid through the central lymphatic system and into the circulatory system. Diaphragmatic breathing may also feel soothing and reduce our stress levels.

Let's learn diaphragmatic breathing:

- Begin in a relaxed yet alert position.
- Place one hand just below your rib cage.
- Breathe in slowly through your nose (or mouth if your nose is blocked) so that your abdomen moves out against your hand.
- Your upper chest should remain relatively still.
- Breathe out through your nose or mouth as your belly button moves in toward the spine.

Let's put diaphragmatic breathing into practice by trying 5 minutes of 5/5 breathing:

- Begin in a relaxed yet alert position. Your eyes can be open or closed.
- Exhale fully.

- Inhale for a count of 5.
- Exhale for a count of 5.
- Repeat for 5 minutes (around 30 breaths total).

Using a breathing app or the stopwatch timer on your phone can help you keep track of your breathing.

Cyclic Sighing

Cyclic sighing consists of taking a two-part deep inhale and a longer exhale. Many people do this naturally during stressful moments. Practicing this type of breathing has been shown to bring psychological relief, and the effects increase with regular practice (Balban et al., 2023).

Let's try cyclic sighing:

- Begin in a relaxed yet alert position. Your eyes can be open or closed.
- Exhale fully.
- Breathe in through your nose.
- When your lungs feel full, take another, shorter inhale through the nose to fully inflate your lungs.
- Exhale slowly.
- Repeat for a total of 3 breaths at first, eventually working up to 5 minutes.

Manual Lymphatic Drainage (MLD) Massage

A few weeks after my drains were removed, I started massaging my face and neck to encourage lymphatic drainage. Manual lymphatic drainage (MLD) massage may reduce swelling after plastic surgery, which is important because "rapidly reducing lymphostasis postoperatively may help improve early results and prevent late sequelae" (Marxen et al., 2023). Lymphostasis is the building up of lymphatic fluid (swelling) in tissues.

MLD is so much more than just a relaxing massage. Researchers have found that "manual lymphatic drainage can be performed to reduce edema and pain as well as enhance the range of motion and patients' quality of life" (Jung et al., 2024). Researchers state that "in addition to fighting this accumulation of fluid, doing lymphatic drainage after plastic surgery may help in recovery, improving blood circulation, reducing pain, and facilitating healing" (Marxen et al., 2023).

What does the research show? Including MLD in your postoperative protocol may result in a reduction in breathlessness and improvement in sleep. MLD can also help our body balance hormone levels by increasing circulation and releasing hormones from edematous tissue, causing "increased urinary secretion of adrenergic hormones, serotonin, and histamine" in people with lymphedema (Marxen et al., 2023).

With your surgeon's permission, try my self-MLD routine for the first weeks after facial plastic surgery. The first video is for the first week or two after surgery. It combines gentle MLD strokes at the bottom of the neck with relaxing diaphragmatic breathing. The second video is for week three and beyond. It combines diaphragmatic breathing, MLD strokes on the face and neck, and neck and shoulder movements to help the lymphatic system drain fluid. Omit the neck movements until your surgeon allows full range of motion in the head and neck.

https://bit.ly/faceliftbreathing

https://bit.ly/faceliftselfmassage

Here is an eight-week breathing and guided meditation video series for plastic surgery recovery:

https://bit.ly/plasticsurgerybreathing

Stress Reduction

Healing from a facelift is a stressful experience. We're so worried about getting it wrong. We're worried about harming ourselves if we sleep wrong or not enough, move wrong or too much, or eat the wrong foods that increase our swelling. Seeing our faces swollen and bruised can bring up strong emotions. All this tension and worry sends stress hormones coursing through our bodies.

Reducing stress is important to getting the best results from a facelift. Researchers have found that chronic stress can "impede wound healing, affecting recovery from plastic surgery and other invasive cosmetic procedures" (Pickart & Margolina, 2018). A chapter titled "Psychological Tools to Assist Your Practice" in the textbook *Essential Psychiatry for the Aesthetic Practitioner* recommends stress reduction techniques, including progressive muscle relaxation and deep abdominal breathing for reducing stress around cosmetic procedures (Rieder & Fried, 2021). We have practiced abdominal breathing already, let's learn about progressive muscle relaxation.

Progressive muscle relaxation is a mind-body practice that uses our muscles to help the body reduce the negative effects of stress. A Progressive Muscle Relaxation protocol consists of contracting different muscle groups for five to seven seconds and then relaxing them for ten seconds. If it's right after your facelift, you can omit the face and neck portion and start at the upper back. REMEMBER: Ask your surgeon before using this practice and don't do anything not cleared by your surgeon!

Progressive Muscle Relaxation (PMR):

- Lie or sit down comfortably in a quiet area where you will not be disturbed.
- Take a few deep breaths, and close your eyes if it makes you more comfortable.
- Squeeze each muscle group for five to seven seconds, then relax for 10 seconds.
- The whole practice should take about 10–15 minutes.

Optional:

- Scrunch your forehead, then relax.
- Squeeze your eyes shut, then relax.
- Scrunch your nose, then relax.
- Purse your lips, then relax.
- Tense all the muscles in your face, then relax.
- Feel the heaviness of your face.

My Alternative:

- Smile, then relax.
- Open the mouth wide or yawn, then relax.
- Pucker up the mouth, then relax.

Body portion:

- Tense the muscles in your shoulders by scrunching your shoulders up, then relax.
- Feel the heaviness of your shoulders.
- Tense all the muscles in your upper torso, then relax.

- Feel the heaviness of your upper torso.
- Tense the muscles in your upper arms, then relax.
- Feel the heaviness of your upper arms.
- Tense the muscles in your forearms, then relax.
- Feel the heaviness of your forearms.
- Tense the muscles in your hands by making fists, then relax.
- Feel the heaviness of your hands.
- Tense the muscles in your fingers, then relax.
- Feel the heaviness of your fingers.
- Tense all the muscles in your arms, then relax.
- Feel the heaviness of your arms.
- Tense the muscles in your abdomen, then relax.
- Feel the heaviness of your abdomen.
- Tense the muscles in your butt, then relax.
- Feel the heaviness of your butt.
- Tense the muscles in your thighs, then relax.
- Feel the heaviness of your thighs.
- Tense the muscles in the front of your lower legs, then relax (lift your toes).
- Feel the heaviness of your lower legs.
- Tense your calf muscles, then relax (point your toes).
- Feel the heaviness of your calves.
- Tense the muscles in your feet, then relax (lift your toes).
- Feel the heaviness of your feet.
- Curl and tense your toes, then relax.
- Feel the heaviness of your toes.

- Tense all the muscles in your legs, then relax.
- Feel the heaviness of your legs.
- Tense all the muscles in your entire body, then relax.
- Feel the heaviness of your entire body.
- Know that you can repeat this practice any time to reduce the stress in your body.
- Take a few deep breaths to transition out of the practice.

Try this PMR practice while you are healing from surgery: https://bit.ly/pmrafterfacelift

Once you are fully healed you can try the full video here:

https://bit.ly/fullpmrafterfacelift

You can also try this 10-minute PMR practice video with audio guidance from Northwestern Medicine: https://bit.ly/PMRNorthwestern

What's happening if these breathing and stress reduction practices don't make you feel relaxed? Many people who have anxiety can experience negative feelings when they try to relax. These feelings are called Relaxation Induced Anxiety (RIA), and may happen because worrying feels safer than relaxing and becoming aware of internal bodily sensations.

It's okay if relaxing our body feels emotionally neutral. We're not 'failing' at relaxing if we don't feel calm and restored. If you're struggling with feeling comfortable relaxing, speaking to a mental health professional may help.

Vibration

Why use vibration to help your recovery from facelift? Vibration is motion, and movement of the tissues after surgery can affect blood flow and drainage from the tissues, helping reduce swelling and inflammation. A researcher found that using a vibrating nasal cast reduced edema and pain after rhinoplasty (Tas, 2020). I didn't use vibration on my nose after my rhinoplasty, but I did use a handheld vibration tool on my face and neck. I started by just gently laying the tool against my skin, then worked up to moving it across my skin in the direction of lymphatic drainage. If you own a vibrating toothbrush, it can be used to apply vibration to the inside of your cheeks and lips. REMEMBER: Ask your surgeon before using vibration and don't use anything not cleared by your surgeon!

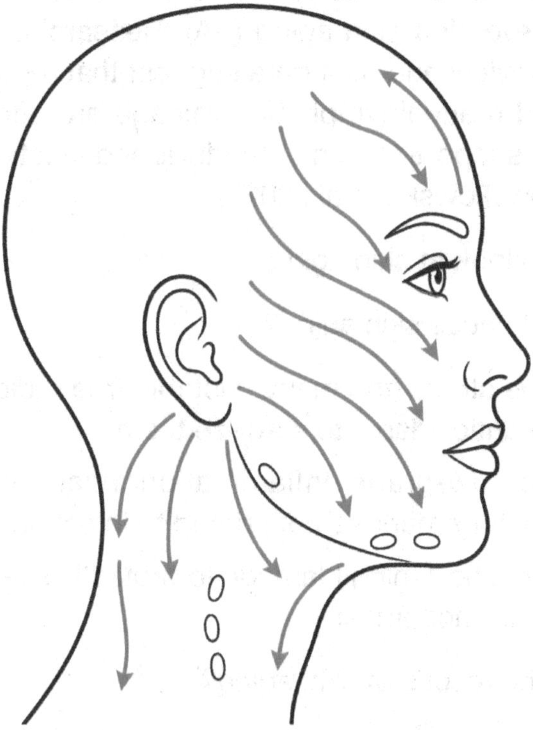

After you have started professional massages, you can try this five minute facial vibration massage protocol: https://bit.ly/vibrationfacemassage

After You are Healed - MLD and Self-Massage

Skin Aging (SA) and MLD

Yes, it's okay to continue receiving lymphatic massage even after you're healed from surgery. Researchers state that "many people undergo facial massages to feel fresh and rejuvenated, tighten the skin, and delay the onset of wrinkles" (Jung et al., 2024). MLD may also help you protect your investment in your face by preventing skin aging (SA). Researchers state that "literature review and pilot data suggest that regular physical activity and manual lymphatic drainage are effective in SA prevention, supporting skin's structural and functional integrity safely" (Nowakowska et al., 2025).

Let's take a look at skin aging.

What might cause skin aging?

- Oxidative stress (too many unstable free radicals and not enough antioxidants to stabilize them)
- Chronic low-grade inflammation/inflammaging (pro-inflammatory markers not related to infection)
- Telomere shortening (damage to protective cap at the end of our chromosomes)

What are the results of skin aging?

- Degradation of collagen fibers (protein that provides structure to tissues)
- Loss of skin firmness and elasticity (wrinkles)
- Discoloration

- Volume loss (looking hollow)

How might lymphatic massage help?

- Enhance tissue drainage
- Reduce swelling
- Affect the tension of fascial structures

(Nowakowska et al., 2025)

How might manual lymphatic drainage massage of the face and neck help after facial rejuvenation surgery? Researchers state that "manual lymphatic drainage (MLD) has been identified as a valuable tool in the management of mature skin. The reduction of swelling, enhancement of microcirculation, and provision of a relaxing effect contribute to the delay of the manifestations of SA by improving its overall appearance and condition" (Nowakowska et al., 2025).

What is the relationship between lymphatic flow and skin health? Researchers have found that "the following improvements have been observed in relation to microcirculation and tissue nourishment: improved lymphatic flow has been demonstrated to positively impact skin health, contributing to enhanced oxygenation and nourishment of skin cells. This, in turn, results in healthier skin tone and increased firmness" (Nowakowska et al., 2025).

Lymphatic massage could be a part of a longevity focused self-care protocol. Researchers caution that it's important to "integrate lymphatic massage with other skincare strategies, such as physical activity, anti-inflammatory diets, or collagen stimulation, to achieve enduring enhancements in skin quality." They explain that "regular use of MLD combined with individually tailored physical activity may be an effective strategy for delaying SA signs and improving overall well-being. It is imperative that interventions are adapted to the individual needs of patients in order to ensure optimal outcomes" (Nowakowska et al., 2025).

Should You Add Face Massage to Your Self-Care Protocol?

Facial massage may be more than just a relaxing experience, it may actually help tissue health. Researchers state that "facial massage is empirically known to induce changes in the facial contours and improve facial sagging." They explain that "facial massage could have tightening and lifting effects, and these would contribute to morphological changes of the face, including the subcutaneous adipose tissue and the SMAS," or superficial musculoaponeurotic system. Why does massage help? They state that "increased blood and lymphatic flow are thought to be the main factors underlying the effectiveness of massages" (Okuda et al., 2022).

Face massage may have both physical and emotional benefits. Researchers state that "interventions that combine visible skin improvements with subjective feelings of care and personalization, such as daily self-massage or tailored at-home regimens, have been shown to positively influence mood, reduce stress, and support emotional well-being" (Haykal et al., 2025b). A different group of researchers also found that two weeks of a three minute face massage resulted in "clinical and self-observed skin benefits, and feelings of well-being" (Flament et al., 2023).

Here is a short facial self-massage video you could perform morning and night once you are healed from your surgery: https://bit.ly/postfaceliftmassage

This video combines the facial self-massage protocol with facial massage rollers: https://bit.ly/faceliftmassageroller

The research study recommending this protocol is at:

https://bit.ly/Okuda2021

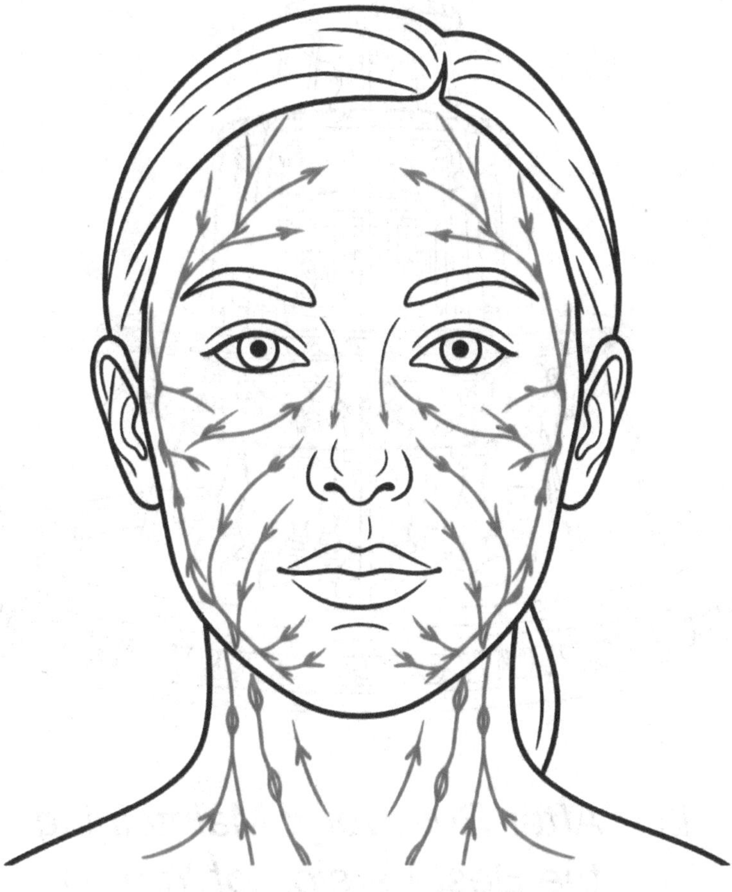

Part Two

Feel as Good as You Look

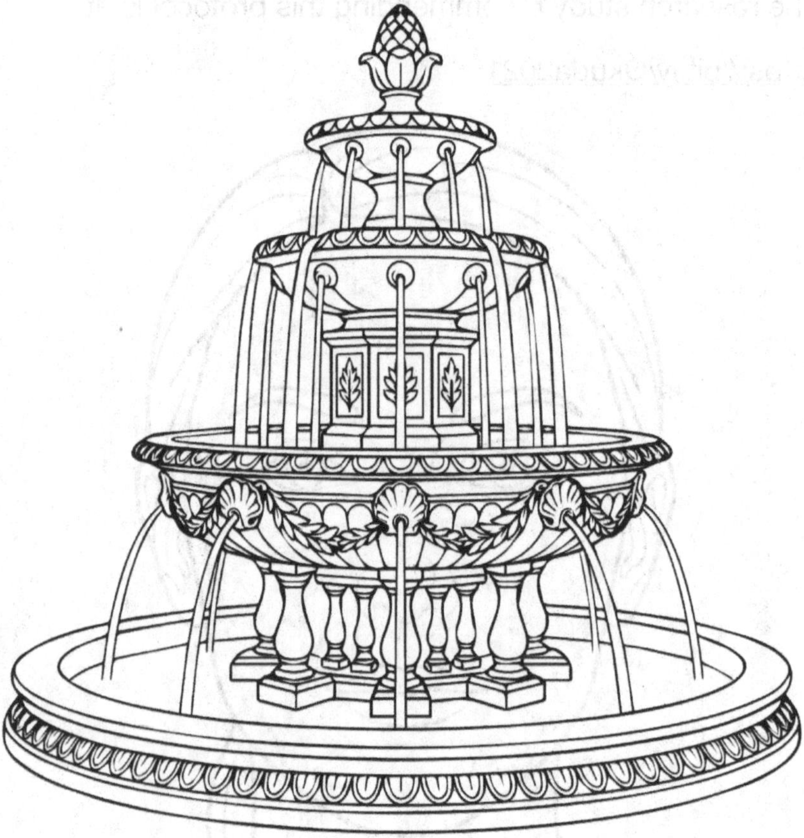

Life After Recovery: Maintaining the Best Version of You

What's Making Us Feel Older?

Earlier, we learned that people get a facelift to improve their quality of life, for personal or professional growth or to boost self-confidence. For me, it was to look as young as I felt inside. Once I had healed and was enjoying my new face and neck, I realized that the goal had now shifted. As I approached menopause, I wanted to stay healthy and keep feeling as young as I now looked in the mirror. I wanted to learn more about longevity and healthspan and give myself the resources I needed to live a long and healthy life.

I will now put on my health coach hat and share some of those resources with you. There's no real 'secret' or fountain of youth. It will be advice you've heard before. The difference is that now we will learn exactly why these healthy self-care behaviors are important as we age. Let's start by looking at some different ways to understand aging.

Lifespan can be split up into four stages: Two when we are young and two when we are older adults. We have all passed through the first two. Researchers share that "old age is often divided into two phases in aging research: the "Third Age," when people are usually active and independent, and the "Fourth Age," which is the last stage of life (and is typically characterized by multimorbidity, functional loss, cognitive decline, motor and sensory impairment, and frailty)" (Turska-Kawa & Pilch, 2025).

How can we enjoy the results of our facial rejuvenation surgery and stay active and independent in our Third Age for as long as possible? When we talk about aging and longevity, first we have to define different types of "aging."

Chronological age is a measurement of time: our actual age in years. We'd need space or time travel to change our chronological age.

Physiological/biological aging measures changes in the body based on certain cellular or molecular parameters. Biological aging CAN be reversed or slowed.

We all know our chronological age is how many birthday candles were on our cake this year. But how can we tell what age we are biologically?

PhenoAge is one way to discover if you have a different biological age than your chronological age. The PhenoAge Biological Age Calculator estimates your biological age using your recent Complete Blood Count (CBC) and Comprehensive Metabolic Panel (CMP) results.

The calculation utilizes lab values of:

- Albumin
- Creatinine
- Glucose
- Serum C-reactive protein
- Lymphocyte percent
- Mean cell volume
- Red cell distribution width
- Alkaline phosphatase
- White blood cell count

(Levine et al., 2018).

I was able to pull up my recent blood work and plug my lab numbers into an online calculator relatively easily. Search online for PhenoAge Biological Age Calculator to find a free calculator. Learn your score, and keep on reading to learn about the link between loneliness and increased PhenoAge later in the book.

Another measurement of health is Optimal Cardiometabolic Health, which is defined in the US as having a:

- BMI <25 kg/m2 AND WC ≤88 cm (women)/WC ≤102 cm (men)
- Blood Glucose - FPG <100 mg/dL AND HbA1c <5.7% AND NOT taking diabetes medication
- Cholesterol TC:HDL under 5:1 AND NOT taking lipid-lowering medication
- Blood pressure: SBP <120 AND DBP <80 AND NOT taking BP-lowering medications
- No history of cardiovascular disease

Why is blood glucose important? Researchers state that chronic high blood sugar can affect blood vessels, and people with increased HbA1c have an increased risk for peripheral arterial disease, even if they don't have diabetes (Guo et al., 2026). Having a high blood glucose level may lead to premature aging of the skin. Researchers found that perceived age increases by over 4 months for every 1 mmol/L increase in average daily glucose level in non-diabetic subjects (Noordam et al., 2013).

BMI can be estimated using online calculators, and the rest of these numbers can be found in the data collected from your last yearly physical. Researchers found that less than 7% of Americans screened in the National Health and Nutrition Examination Survey in 2017-2018 had optimal cardiometabolic health. Read more about this study: https://pmc.ncbi.nlm.nih.gov/articles/PMC10475326/

Two other important concepts are lifespan and healthspan.

- Lifespan is the total amount of time we are alive.
- Healthspan is the amount of time we are free of serious chronic illness and disability that affect our ability to complete activities of daily living.

It's relatively easy to begin increasing lifespan. We don't have to understand chemistry, reconstitute peptides, or give up on our responsibilities. We just have to start making small changes in three key areas.

Researchers found that focusing on SPAN behaviors of sleep, physical activity, and nutrition (SPAN) can improve longevity. Specifically, sleeping for ten more minutes, increasing moderate to vigorous physical activity by five minutes per day, and eating an extra quarter cup of vegetables per day may result in a ten percent decrease in risk of major adverse cardiovascular events (MACE), including heart attack and stroke (Koemel et al., 2026).

What is the next step after we have succeeded in consistently making these changes? The optimal SPAN protocol is associated with 57% lower risk of MACE:

- 8.0–9.5 h/day sleep
- 40–105 min/day moderate to vigorous physical activity
- Dietary Quality Score (DQS) 33–50

(Koemel et al., 2026).

The researchers' DQS emphasizes a higher intake of vegetables, fruits, fish, dairy, whole grains, and vegetable oils and a lower intake of refined grains, processed meats, unprocessed red meats, and sugar-sweetened beverages (Koemel et al., 2026).

Like I said, there's no new advice here, it's everything we've been hearing from doctors for decades. No unusual blood tests or fanatical protocols are needed to start increasing lifespan.

Let's look at healthspan now.

Healthspan describes the absence of chronic disease and disability. The important difference between healthspan and lifespan is why we actually have two different ways to measure our life: life expectancy and health-adjusted life expectancy. Researchers share that "the difference in life expectancy and health-adjusted life expectancy (i.e., healthspan-lifespan gap) represents the number of years lived with disease or disability" (Garmany & Terzic, 2024).

Unfortunately, there is a huge gap between when people die and when they start losing quality of life due to disability. Researchers state that "the gap between lifespan (total years lived) and healthspan (years free from diseases) is approximately nine years worldwide" (Wang et al., 2025). A gap of almost a decade is already troubling, but unfortunately, the United States has an even larger gap. Research has found that "the US presented the largest healthspan-lifespan gap, amounting to 12.4 years, underpinned by a rise in noncommunicable diseases" (Garmany & Terzic, 2024). That is what I refer to as the difficult dozen—many Americans will spend their last twelve years losing their quality of life, independence, and health due to disease and disability.

Healthspan worries are a big reason why many people may be hesitant to live to be ninety or a hundred. For many people, increased lifespan isn't desirable if our final extra years aren't pleasant.

Participants in a study from Singapore "emphasised that their desired lifespan was contingent on several factors, such as maintaining cognitive function, avoiding being housebound, and not becoming a burden to others. The importance of quality of life was a recurrent theme" (Wang et al., 2025).

Gender may have a role in how we live in our old age, and women's lives may end differently than men's. In Italy, "while women tend to live longer, in the last five years of life, they often experience diseases and disability" and "men facing health problems are more likely to succumb to those problems compared to women with similar health issues" (Candore et al., 2024).

Healthspan ends when we need assistance with activities of daily living or when chronic illnesses put us in poor health and reduce our quality of life. The good news is that physical activity can help increase our healthspan.

How can we find out whether our healthspan is at risk? Researchers from Yale University found that a declining score on a Short Physical Performance Battery (SPPB) was the strongest risk factor for eventual disability in a study of people over seventy years old (Gill et al., 2009). Research published in the *New England Journal of Medicine* found that adults over seventy who performed poorly on a functional assessment had a higher risk of disability in the future. The assessment included a standing balance test, timed walk, and a sit to stand challenge (Guralnick et al., 1995).

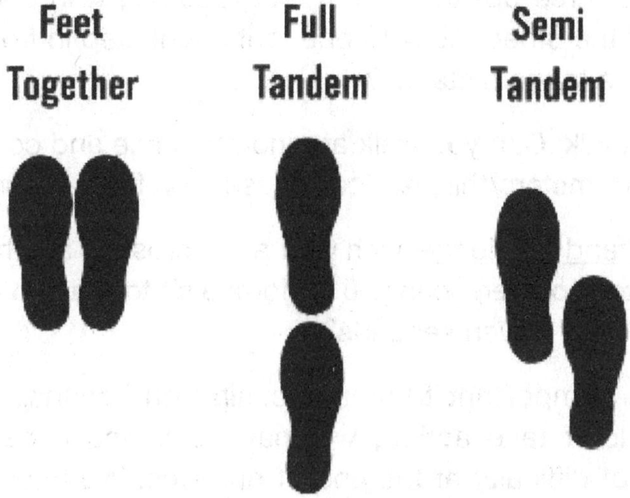
Feet
Together
Full
Tandem
Semi
Tandem

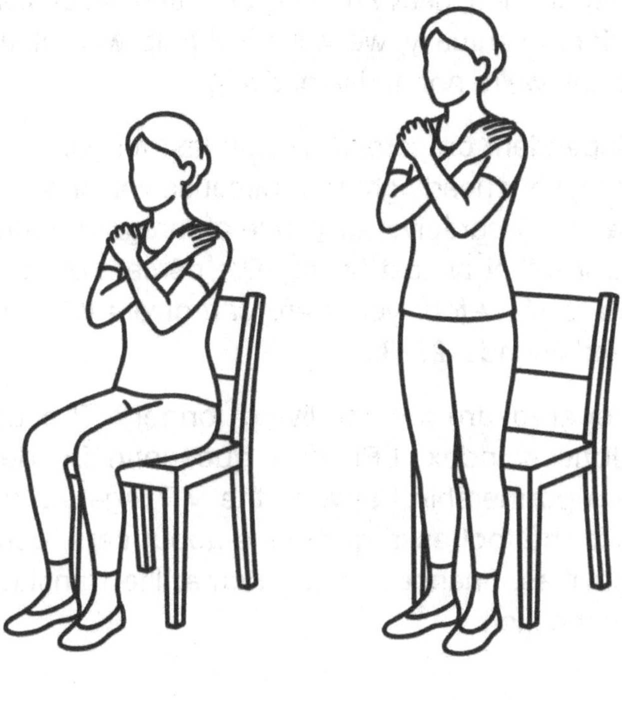

Standing Balance: Can you stand for longer than ten seconds in these three positions: with feet together, with one foot in front of the other and with one foot a half step in front of the other in a tandem stance?

Timed Walk: Can you walk at a normal pace and cover more than four meters/thirteen feet in less than five seconds?

Sit to Stand Challenge: with your arms crossed and hands on opposite shoulders, can you perform a sit-to-stand movement five times in eleven seconds?

Why is it important to start focusing on healthspan now? If we don't take action, we may be facing a decade or longer of difficulty at the end of our lives. We may lose our independence, having to rely on others to help us. First, we will stop exercising and slow down. Then, we will need help with transportation, heavy housework, medications, and meal preparation. Eventually, we will need help with all activities, even though we're not at risk of dying.

Being dependent on caregivers can last for years. You may be nodding your head right now because you know someone who is a family caregiver or you're a caregiver yourself. The CDC reports that almost twenty-five percent of adults aged forty-five to sixty-four years are caregivers (Caregiving for Family and Friends, 2018).

How prepared are we for living longer? The Longevity Preparedness Index (LPI) is a questionnaire developed through a partnership between the MIT AgeLab and John Hancock. The tool asks questions about care, community, daily activities, finance, health, home, life transitions, and social connection.

Find your score here: https://www.johnhancock.com/ideas-insights/longevity-preparedness-index.html

The tests mentioned above can give us a good idea of our biological age, risk for cardiovascular disease, frailty, and how prepared we are to live a long and healthy life. I hope your results inspire you to continue to focus on self-care after you are healed from your facelift surgery.

Ten Longevity Concepts

As you begin to read more about longevity, you may come across terms like inflammaging and oxidative stress and hear about the importance of epigenetics, gut microbiome, mitochondria, and telomeres. Don't give up! Longevity is an absolutely huge topic, but we don't need to get a degree in medicine to figure out how to stay healthy. Let's start with just focusing on ten concepts about longevity and holistic self-care practices that address each concept.

These topics might give you the basis for a good beginner's self-care routine as you recover from your facelift. Remember, we learned earlier that physical activity is good for skin health and that oxidative stress, inflammaging, and telomere shortening have an impact on skin aging, including loss of skin firmness and elasticity (Nowakowska et al., 2025).

1. The Difficult Dozen

We know the three most common diseases that end lifespan: cardiovascular disease, cancers and neurological disorders. Let's learn what's ending healthspan and contributing to what I call the Difficult Dozen—the twelve years of pain in between the end of healthspan and the end of lifespan.

Researchers point a finger toward "mental and substance use disorders, along with musculoskeletal diseases" as having contributed most to years lived with disability in the US. For women, the burden is mostly due to "musculoskeletal, genitourinary, and neurological diseases" when compared to men (Garmany & Terzic, 2024). Musculoskeletal conditions affect joints, muscles, bones (including the spine), ligaments and tendons, including low back pain, neck pain, and arthritis. Research has found that "back and neck pain present the world's largest disease burden related to years lived with disability" (Diez et al., 2022).

The good news is that massage is a commonly used treatment for symptoms of musculoskeletal conditions and is most often used for back pain and chronic pain (Ladanyi et al., 2025). A combination of exercise and routine massage may be an excellent way to reduce the negative effects of back and neck pain (Reynolds et al., 2025) (Narenthiran et al., 2025). And yes, of course a massage therapist would recommend regular massage for keeping ourselves happy and active as we age. I receive regular massages and so should you.

Now, let's look at what else is important.

<u>Reducing the Difficult Dozen - Lifestyle Changes for Longevity and Healthspan</u>

If you're interested in staying healthy, you won't be surprised to read that diet and exercise have a big impact on both health and longevity. Specifically, researchers state that "a combination of the correct dose of physical activity, an appropriate gut microbiota, and genetic predisposition, together with an antioxidant-rich diet, is the key for successful aging" (Deledda et al., 2022).

The focus is NOT on 'getting skinny' or just 'eating less and moving more,' like a lot of dieting advice we've heard. Longevity advice seems to be focused on:

- Physical activity
- Gut microbiota
- Epigenetics (lifestyle habits)
- Antioxidants as a part of a healthy diet

We will dive into information on these keys to successful aging throughout this section. Let's look at epigenetics first.

Epigenetics and Longevity

Yes, how long we will live is partly dependent upon our DNA, but epigenetics also has a role, and we can take actions that may influence our epigenetics. Researchers state that "epigenetics plays a crucial role in the aging process by regulating gene expression without altering DNA sequences. Factors such as environmental exposure, diet, and lifestyle choices influence epigenetic modifications, which can accelerate or decelerate aging" (Haykal et al., 2025). Lifestyle choices, like what we eat, how we exercise, stress reduction, quality sleep, our social ties, and exposure to pollutants in the environment, may alter gene expression without changing our DNA. All these positive self-care habits might influence our epigenetics.

2. Blue Zones

Blue Zones Research and Longevity

What might successful nutrition, exercise, and lifestyle habits look like in real life? Certain areas in the world have a large percentage of people living long and healthy lives. We call these special communities 'Blue Zones.' Researchers have found that these Blue Zones are "regions of the world that have a higher number of individuals who live longer than the expected average" (Kreouzi et al., 2024). Researchers examined lifestyles in these communities and found many similarities, which they call Blue Zone principles.

Blue Zone Principles include:

- Moving naturally
- Eating wisely
- Improving resilience to stress
- Getting adequate sleep
- Keeping strong family ties
- Community support
- Respect for the planet
- Having a purpose in life

(Kreouzi et al., 2024).

Not surprisingly, these principles are similar in some ways to the Six Pillars of Lifestyle Medicine:

- Healthy eating
- Exercising
- Avoiding smoking tobacco and other risky substances
- Stress management
- Restorative sleep
- Forming and maintaining relationships

(Kreouzi et al., 2024).

This is all common advice for leading a healthy life. But just because they sound like common sense doesn't mean they're actually making us healthier. What are these lifestyle interventions actually trying to change in the body and mind to enhance longevity?

In order to find out, we'll have to define aging again, this time in a more medical way. Researchers share that "aging is a multifactorial process that includes numerous mechanisms, such as the shortening of telomeres, systemic inflammation, oxidative stress, and a deficiency of cellular energy, mainly due to autophagy and mitochondrial dysfunction, causing cells to enter a state of senescence and cellular cycle arrest" (Salehi et al., 2020). Autophagy is the process of "digesting useless components and those that work improperly in cells" (Yegorov et al., 2020). Senescence is the process of growing old/aging.

Wow, that's a "multifactorial process," indeed. Let's break it down:

- Systemic inflammation
- Mitochondrial dysfunction
- Telomere shortening
- Oxidative stress

Taking action and making nutrition, exercise, and other lifestyle changes might benefit our body by protecting our telomeres and reducing systemic inflammation, oxidative stress, and mitochondrial dysfunction. If there are healthy habits I can build that have been shown to do one or more of these things, I'm interested in learning more!

We have learned that keeping a healthy lifestyle may be important for living a long life. Now, let's dive deeper into the effects of inflammation, mitochondria, telomeres, and oxidative stress on longevity.

3. Inflammation

Inflammation and Longevity

Inflammation may have a role both in healing from facial plastic surgery and our overall health. Researchers state that “the skin’s immune system plays a significant role in aging and tissue repair. Chronic low-grade inflammation, often referred to as “inflammaging,” contributes to tissue breakdown and delayed wound healing. This persistent inflammation state disrupts the skin barrier, accelerates collagen degradation, and impairs the skin’s ability to repair itself efficiently” (Haykal et al., 2025).

Reducing inflammation and ‘inflammaging’ may be an important part of keeping our skin looking younger after facelift and necklift, and it may also help our body as well. Inflammation has an effect on many systems in the body, and “low-grade inflammation is increasingly recognized as a shared characteristic of metabolic, psychiatric, and neurodegenerative diseases” (Chavda et al., 2024).

What lifestyle factors might we change to limit low-level chronic inflammation? Researchers share that “smoking, diet, sedentary lifestyle, obesity, hormones, stress, and irregular sleep patterns” are all causes of inflammation (Chavda et al., 2024), so smoking cessation, a nutritious diet, a healthy level of exercise, and improving sleep may help reduce chronic inflammation levels. Stress reduction practices may also help. Look for stress reduction practices that may have an effect on inflammatory cytokines. Research shows that by “modulating the activity of pro-inflammatory cytokines such as interleukin-6 (IL- 6) and tumor necrosis factor- alpha (TNF- α) … therapies aim to reduce chronic inflammation and restore homeostasis in the skin microenvironment” (Haykal et al., 2025).

Breathwork for Beauty

A twenty-minute breathing practice taken from the Thirumanthiram, an ancient medical text from India, has been shown to reduce several stress and inflammatory biomarkers (Twal et al., 2016). The protocol includes OM/AUM chanting and thirumoolar pranayamam (TMP).

Watch one of the coauthors share these practices in this video: https://bit.ly/ThirumoolarPranayama

If you are healed from surgery, let's try the protocol! Sit in a comfortable yet alert position with a straight spine, and close your eyes if that feels comfortable.

First:

- Inhale deeply through both nostrils.
- Exhale slowly while chanting OM/AUM.
- Repeat for 10 minutes.

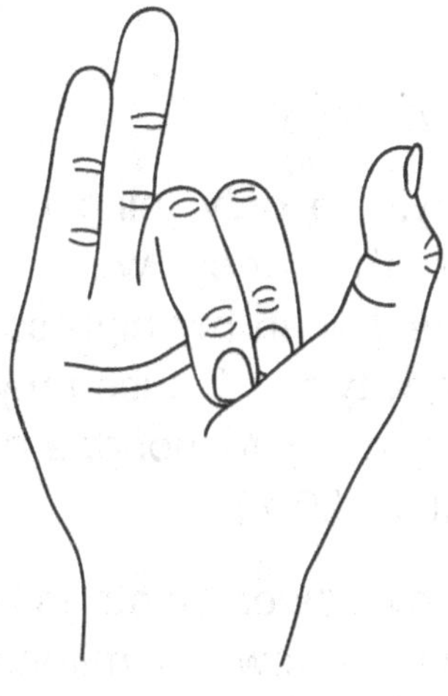

Vishnu Mudra

Then:

- Hold your right hand in Vishnu mudra/Mrigi Mudra (index and middle finger held at the base of the thumb) to help you close off each nostril when needed.
- Close your right nostril with your right thumb and inhale through your left nostril, silently repeating the phrase "I'm relaxed" twice.
- Close both nostrils and hold the breath while silently repeating the phrase "I'm relaxed" eight times.
- Keep your ring finger on your left nostril and release your thumb. Exhale through your right nostril while silently repeating the phrase "I'm relaxed" four times.
- Repeat this cycle for 10 minutes.
- Take a few deep breaths through both nostrils before ending the practice.

(Balasubramanian, 2015).

4. Mitochondria

<u>Mitochondria and Longevity</u>

Before I turned fifty, the only thing I remembered about mitochondria was that they were described as the 'powerhouses of the cell' in my high school biology class. Learning about longevity has focused my interest on how to improve the health of my mitochondria because of their role in aging (Candore et al., 2024).

Why might these tiny power plants inside our cells be so important? Researchers now call mitochondria "the pivotal players in the aging process." When mitochondria become dysfunctional, the cell suffers from "reduced oxidative capacity and a consequent increase in oxidative damage," which lead to biological aging (Deledda et al., 2022).

Mitochondria may have a direct effect on our skin health after facelift and necklift. Having well-functioning mitochondria affects "energy production, oxidative stress, and skin regeneration. Recent research has shown that mitochondrial dysfunction contributes to the breakdown of collagen and elastin, leading to premature aging" and mitochondria affect "photoprotection, homeostasis, and overall skin longevity" (Haykal et al., 2025).

How might we support our mitochondria? One way is to practice gratitude in the evening. Researchers found that people with a positive attitude in the evening also had higher mitochondrial health (Picard et al., 2018). We can practice gratitude by keeping a gratitude journal. I suggest using pen and paper. Make your first goal to write at least five sentences about one thing you are grateful for each night. Begin slowly by journaling several times a week and work up to a daily practice. Later, you can expand your gratitude journal to also record three to five things for which you are grateful on a daily basis. Think back over your day and include anything, however small or great, that was a source of gratitude that day. Make the list personal, and try to think of different things each day.

Tips for keeping a gratitude journal

- <u>Be specific</u> - focus on the details of why and how the things in your life inspire gratitude.
- <u>Go in depth</u> - Spend a little time focusing on each item in the day's journal entry.
- <u>Focus on people as well as things</u> - Remember to also focus on people for whom you are grateful.

- Keep it simple - You don't need a fancy journal or a timer to start practicing gratitude journaling.
- Make it a habit - Set aside a time and place to write in your journal if it's proving hard to adopt as a habit.
- Don't make it a source of guilt - Feeling gratitude shouldn't feel forced or make you feel guilty or ashamed. Some of us are embarrassed by loved ones and called 'ungrateful' when we try to advocate for our needs. Gratitude shouldn't feel manipulative.

Exercise may also help mitochondrial health. Research has shown that "physical activity is linked to improved mitochondrial function, and importantly, represents a mechanism for the potential reversal of decline in adults" (Boon et al., 2025).

What type of exercise might build healthy mitochondria? Research states that "heart rate zones 1 and 2 are zones in which mitochondria utilize fatty acids—the preferred fuel (substrate) for optimal mitochondrial function. Zones 1 and 2 are not difficult and allow a person to carry on a conversation while walking. As one's endurance increases, the resting heart rate decreases and indirect maximal oxygen consumption (VO2Max) increases, enabling one to experience the benefits firsthand and know that they are achieving mitochondrial fitness" (Boon et al., 2025). We will learn how to monitor VO2Max later in this section.

Strength training may also improve mitochondrial health. Resistance exercises may improve health because "sarcopenia, the age-related decline in muscle mass and function, poses a significant health challenge as the global population ages. Mitochondrial dysfunction is a key factor in sarcopenia, as evidenced by the role of mitochondrial reactive oxygen species (mtROS) in mitochondrial biogenesis and dynamics, as well as mitophagy. Resistance exercise training (RET) is a well-established intervention for sarcopenia" (Jeong et al., 2024).

5. Telomeres

Telomeres and Longevity

What are telomeres? Telomeres are at the end of our DNA in chromosomes. Unfortunately, "telomeres, which are essential for genomic stability, naturally shorten with cell division." Every time a cell replicates, the telomeres shorten. Research has found that "telomere shortening, which is accelerated by stress, inflammation, and oxidative damage, is linked to age-related diseases, such as cardiovascular disorders, cancer, and neurodegenerative conditions" (Giridharan, 2024). Telomere length can be affected by oxidative stress and lifestyle choices (Boccardi, 2025). When telomeres become too short to do their job of protecting the chromosome's DNA, the result is cellular aging, increased risk of mutation, senescence, and cell death (Everly & Ramirez, 2025).

Research has found that "the regulation of the length and function of telomeres is an important factor in maintaining health and longevity" (Salehi et al., 2020). What might we do to protect our telomeres? A study found that comprehensive lifestyle changes (diet, activity, stress management, and social support) were associated with increased relative telomere length, even five years later (Ornish, 2013).

How might we care for our telomeres? Mindfulness and yoga are two options. Research has found that "mindfulness interventions significantly affect ... age-related DNA telomere maintenance activity" (Diez et al., 2022). Research has also shown that regular practice of the asana, pranayama, and meditation arms of yoga may result in "significant improvements in telomere length." Yoga practice can affect oxidative stress, chronic inflammation, immune regulation, mitochondrial health, and telomere dynamics. Research has found that, "yoga and meditation boost cellular resilience by lowering stress, inflammation, and oxidative damage and enhancing neuroendocrine regulation." Practicing yoga and meditation may reduce stress biomarkers, lower inflammatory markers, and enhance telomerase activity (Giridharan, 2024).

6. Oxidative Stress

Oxidative Stress and Longevity

Oxidative stress occurs when there are more free radicals than antioxidants in the body. If there aren't enough antioxidants donating electrons to the free radicals, these radicals steal electrons from nearby molecules, which can result in damage to chromosomes and telomeres, reduction in the body's ability to fight tumors, and cellular death. Smoking, alcohol consumption, pollution, and excessive stress can increase free radicals (Everly & Ramirez, 2025). Antioxidants include vitamin A, vitamin C, vitamin E, lycopene, selenium, and beta-carotene, but just taking a supplement isn't proven to improve lifespan.

Mindfulness practices like Heartfulness Meditation may help the body reduce oxidative stress. A Heartfulness meditation practice includes "relaxation," "cleaning," and "heartfulness prayer" (Patil et al., 2024). Find a sample heartfulness Meditation here: https://bit.ly/beginnerheartfulness

Scientists from the University of Ljubljana's Laboratory for Oxidative Stress Research in Slovenia recommend regular moderate exercise, quality sleep, taking time for relaxation and hobbies, and avoiding excessive psychophysical stress as strategies for reducing oxidative stress (Poljsak, 2011). Other research has found that resistance exercise may also reduce oxidative stress (Jeong et al., 2024).

Quality sleep may be important for reducing oxidative stress. Researchers have found that "sleep optimization is crucial for skin barrier recovery, as deep sleep facilitates growth hormone secretion and reduces cortisol-driven inflammation" (Haykal et al., 2025).

Sleep tape may be one method for improving sleep, especially if you have obstructive sleep apnea (OSA). Research has found that "mouth-taping during sleep improved snoring and the severity of sleep apnea in mouth-breathers with mild OSA" and apnea/hypopnea index (AHI) as well as median snoring index (SI) were reduced by about half. Researchers concluded that "mouth-taping could be an alternative treatment in patients with mild OSA before turning to CPAP therapy or surgical intervention" (Lee et al., 2022).

Deep breathing may help reduce oxidative stress. Let's practice diaphragmatic breathing again to remember the benefits of this practice:

- Begin in a relaxed yet alert position.
- Place one hand just below your rib cage.
- Breathe in slowly through your nose (or mouth if you cannot breathe through your nose) so that your abdomen moves out against your hand.
- Your upper chest should remain relatively still.
- Breathe out through your nose or mouth as your belly button moves in toward the spine.
- Repeat for one minute.

We just learned about the possible negative effects of inflammation and oxidative stress on longevity and the importance of taking care of our mitochondria and telomeres. Now let's look at the importance of reducing stress and building community.

7. Stress Reduction

Stress and Aging

Chronic stress may have an effect on the way we age. Our body's stress response helps protect us from danger or prepare us to achieve important goals. The problem may begin when stress becomes chronic and our stress hormones begin having negative effects on our health. Researchers explain that "the stress response is an adaptive mechanism that allows mobilizing all the resources of the body to fight a temporary threat. When the process becomes chronic, the stress associated with adaptive mechanisms becomes destructive" (Yegorov et al., 2020).

"People exposed to chronic stress age rapidly"

(Yegorov et al., 2020)

The results of chronic stress may open the door to many diseases. Chronic stress may have an effect on inflammation and 'inflammaging.' This affects longevity because research has shown that "inflammaging can contribute to atherosclerosis, diabetes, hypertension" (Yegorov et al., 2020).

Inflammaging may happen when:

- anti-inflammatory cytokines levels decrease

- pro-inflammatory cytokines (interleukin-1 (IL-1), IL-6, tumor necrosis factor alpha (TNF-α), and others) increase
- Innate immune response is altered

(Yegorov et al., 2020).

Cortisol and Aging

There is a correlation between biological aging and cortisol, which is a stress hormone (Wang et al., 2025a). Is cortisol to blame for wrinkles, too? Researchers found that people under moderate stress had "significantly increased signs of microrelief alterations (skin texture and fine lines)" (Pujos et al., 2025). Stress reduction practices may help mitigate these effects. Research has found that "mindfulness interventions significantly affect cortisol levels" (Diez et al., 2022). Two mindfulness techniques are self-soothing touch and yoga nidra.

Receiving hugs and practicing self-soothing touch may also help reduce cortisol levels after a stressful situation. The next time you feel judged, hug a loved one or place a hand over your heart and rub lightly in a circle for twenty seconds while taking a few deep, soothing breaths. Research has shown that this simple action of self-care can lower cortisol levels (Dreisoerner et al., 2021).

Yoga nidra is a guided meditation stress management technique that can reduce cortisol (Moszeik et al., 2025). Researchers have found that practicing yoga nidra might improve sleep quality and reduce stress in participants undergoing cancer treatment (Giridharan, 2024a).

A yoga nidra session includes the following steps:

- Getting comfortable
- Setting an intention

- Body scan
- Breath awareness
- Feeling sensations in the body
- Mental visualizations
- Repeating the intention
- Ending the meditation

Try a yoga nidra session by following the guided meditation in these videos:

Yoga Nidra for Facelift Recovery video: https://bit.ly/yoganidrafacelift

Yoga Nidra for Longevity video:
https://bit.ly/yoganidralongevity

8. Community

Community and Longevity

For some people, recovery from plastic surgery is the first time they experience having to depend on their friends and loved ones. People we thought would be there for us become distant, while casual friends step up and show their support. Other people choose to isolate themselves from friends during their recovery from plastic surgery.

Our outlook on life may affect how long we live as well as our quality of life. Research has found that "psychological factors are amongst the most robust predictors of healthspan and longevity" and "social isolation and overall mental well-being are recognized to be major contributors to all-cause mortality and certain health conditions" (Faria et al., 2024).

We can't focus only on our physical well-being; we also need to focus on mental well-being. Research has found that "loneliness, sleep, boredom, and happiness can have a powerful impact on longevity" (Faria et al., 2024). Our quality of life now can positively affect our length of life later.

One important part of quality of life is social connection. It's so important to longevity that some of the tools measuring age include data on human connection in their calculations. A study that used the PhenoAge found that loneliness and social isolation can affect biological aging in older people (Wang et al., 2026). The Longevity Preparedness Index (LPI) we looked at earlier mentions social connection as one of the main domains of life.

Let's look at some ways to use social connection and community to improve our longevity.

<u>Social Networks, Community Service and Longevity</u>

One of my favorite activities is volunteering with the Caregiver Coalition of San Diego. Volunteering brings benefits to our community as well as health benefits to the volunteers themselves. Research shows that "volunteering as an intervention in itself is supported by clear health benefits to the volunteer, particularly improved mental health and reduced mortality." It's important to donate your time for the right reasons. Benefits were only seen "for those who volunteered for other-oriented reasons" (Nichol et al., 2024).

Volunteering may reduce depression and provide benefits to:

- Physical functioning
- Well-being
- Quality of life

- Pride and empowerment
- Motivation
- Self-efficacy
- Life satisfaction
- Positive affect
- Social support
- Connectedness and community

(Nichol et al., 2024).

Motivation was mentioned in the list above. Motivation and purpose may be important for longevity. Research found that “purposeful individuals lived longer than non-purposeful individuals” and “motivation and purpose in older individuals is positively associated with the maintenance of physical function” (Kreouzi et al., 2024).

We also saw social support, connectedness and community mentioned in the list above. Volunteering can help us build a strong social network. Having friends as we grow older is important, and new friends are much harder to make than they were when we were young and always making pals on the playground or at sports. Friendships may actually make us healthier. Research finds that “older adults with close social ties are more likely to engage in health-promoting behaviors, adhere to medical treatments, and experience lower levels of frailty and cognitive decline” (Aliberti & Capunzo, 2025).

We see strong social connections and purpose as part of the Blue Zones. Lifelong friendships and having a purpose in life are integral parts of cultures that foster longevity.

In the Okinawan lifestyle:

- The social support networks called "Moai" help emotional well-being
- The concept of having a purpose or "Ikigai" helps psychological resilience and purpose

In the Costa Rica blue zone:

- The sense of purpose, known as "plan de vida" is a part of the cultural identity

(Aliberti & Capunzo, 2025).

Purpose, Attitude and Longevity

One of the most interesting things I've learned about longevity is the effect that our viewpoint on our own aging has on our lifespan. If we have a better attitude about aging, we may actually end up living longer. Research shows that "positive perceptions of aging and a positive outlook on life are associated with positive health outcomes and reduced mortality" (Brown et al., 2025).

Having a negative attitude about our own aging may also affect our health. Researchers warn that "the opposite relationship also exists, with an older perceived age being a risk factor for depressive symptoms and physical morbidity. Older adults with more negative self-perceptions related to aging (i.e., higher levels of perceived uselessness) also had increased mortality" (Brown et al., 2025). Volunteering helps us to stay useful to others in our community.

Religion and Longevity

Fostering spirituality may also be an important part of wellness, and community is an important part of spirituality.

Researchers state that "spirituality can be understood as a social determinant of health... spirituality includes a sense of ultimate meaning, purpose, transcendence and connectedness" (Teut et al., 2025).

Practicing your religion may also increase your longevity. A study of over 74,000 women found that "attending a religious service more than once per week was associated with 33% lower all-cause mortality compared with women who had never attended religious services." Researchers concluded that "frequent attendance at religious services was associated with significantly lower risk of all-cause, cardiovascular, and cancer mortality among women" (Li et al., 2016).

We now know why reducing stress and building community are important parts of a longevity lifestyle. Let's finish by looking at the two most popular longevity topics—diet and exercise.

9. Digestion

Digestion and Longevity

Tummy issues often take center stage after a long surgery like a facelift. The combination of anesthesia, pain medications, antibiotics, and reduced exercise can result in constipation and an unhappy digestive system. For a lot of people, digestive problems after surgery are a powerful reminder of how important good digestion is to overall happiness. I remember feeling bloated and anxious, wondering when I would be able to poop again.

Stool softeners and laxatives should only be used on a temporary basis. If digestive problems persist, it's important to focus on gut health. Abdominal massage may benefit the digestive system by stimulating peristalsis, stimulating digestive enzyme secretion, and reducing constipation. Nutrition and exercise may also have an impact the digestive system.

Let's look at our microbiome and how what we eat and how we move can affect our longevity. Microbiome is a term for all the microorganisms that live in our body, and dysbiosis is a term for an imbalance in our microbiome. Dysbiosis may have a role in "age-related conditions such as cardiovascular disease, neurodegeneration, diabetes, and systemic inflammation" (Aliberti & Capunzo, 2025).

There may be a link between aging and changes to the microbiome. Researchers have found that "aging is typically associated with reduced microbiome diversity, characterized by a decline in beneficial bacteria (e.g., Bifidobacterium and Lactobacillus) and an increase in pro-inflammatory species (Firmicutes and Proteobacteria). This shift contributes to "inflammaging," which is chronic low-grade inflammation that accelerates atherosclerosis, insulin resistance, cognitive decline. Gut dysbiosis also weakens intestinal barrier integrity, allowing endotoxins like lipopolysaccharides (LPS) to enter the bloodstream and exacerbate systemic inflammation" (Aliberti & Capunzo, 2025).

The foods we eat can have an impact on gut health. Many cultures include fermented foods in their traditional ways of eating. As a child, we had sauerkraut at special family dinners. My husband's family in India have yogurt as a side dish at meals. Researchers state that "fermented foods such as yogurt, kefir, and kimchi introduce beneficial microbes, further promoting gut health" (Aliberti & Capunzo, 2025).

Having a high fiber diet can also lead to a more diverse gut microbial population. Researchers found that "fiber interventions including inulin and gala-oligosaccharides often report an increase of *Bifidobacterium* and *Lactobacillus* taxa" (Rodriguez et al., 2024). Garlic, leeks, onions, and asparagus are sources of inulin (Smith et al., 2015), and dairy and legumes are sources of gala-oligosaccharides.

What types of bacteria may be beneficial for health, and why? Researchers state that "short-chain fatty acid (SCFA) initiates enterocyte proliferation and mucin secretion, which greatly impact the tightness of the intestinal barrier. SCFAs are produced by bacteria from the genera *Clostridium*, *Eubacterium*, *Fusobacterium*, *Butyrivvibrio, Megasphera*, *Roseburia*, *Feacalibacterium*, and *Eubacterium*" (Dziewiecka et al., 2022).

<u>Exercise Impact on Digestive System and Longevity</u>

Exercise may help our gut microbiome. Researchers found that "the level of physical activity modulates the gastrointestinal microbiota in humans" (Dziewiecka et al., 2022). How does the microbiome change? Researchers found that "compared with ordinary elderly people, elderly athletes have more beneficial bacteria and fewer harmful bacteria in their intestines, which means that long-term exercise training may help to resist gastrointestinal health damage caused by aging" (Li et al., 2025).

Which type of exercise may be best? Research found that "moderate exercise has a beneficial effect on intestinal permeability, absorption and assimilation of electrolytes and nutrients, and on the rate of excretion of toxic metabolic products" (Dziewiecka et al., 2022).

More intense exercise isn't better for health when it comes to our digestive system. Researchers state that "the well-known positive health effects of exercise may be mediated by its beneficial modifications to the gut microbiota. However, when there is an exercise overload, these possible beneficial effects are overweighed by increased intestinal permeability and oxidative stress, promoting inflammation and a catabolic state that negatively impacts the functionality of skeletal muscle" (Dziewiecka et al., 2022). Moderate levels of exercise may help gut microbiota while causing less oxidative stress and inflammation than extended and excessively intense bouts of activity.

Gentle exercise like Qigong may provide benefits to our digestion. Researchers found that "the intervention of Wuqinxi exercise could effectively improve the symptoms of patients. Therefore, the authors believe that long-term Wuqinxi exercise can improve the structure of the host's gut microbiota and alleviate the patient's metabolic syndrome" (Li et al., 2025).

What's specifically may be happening to the gut microbiome during exercise? Research has shown that "moderate-intensity exercise does not affect the diversity of the gut microbiota but impacts its composition, with an increased abundance of SCFA and lactic acid producers, also increasing the relative abundance of *Akkermansia muciniphila* and *Oscillospira*. These observations confirm the positive impact of moderate exercise on the diversity and function of the intestinal microbiota" (Dziewiecka et al., 2022). *Akkermansia muciniphila* is beneficial for the body in several ways, including regulating brain-gut axis signaling (Yuan et al., 2026).

10. Exercise

Exercise and Longevity

I have saved the best topic for last, because exercise may be one of the most valuable ways to stay feeling young. Indeed, muscles may be the 'organ of longevity.'

Why is building muscle so important as we age? Research has found that "loss of muscle mass in older adults is associated not only with falls and fractures but also with an increased risk of chronic diseases such as diabetes, hypertension, heart disease, and cancer" (Jeong et al., 2024).

Our body composition may change as we age. Researchers have found that "aging is associated with muscle loss, increased body fat, reduced bone density, and cardiovascular and cognitive decline, all of which heighten frailty and fall risk" (Aliberti & Capunzo, 2025). I have definitely found it harder to add muscle as I have gotten older.

Exercise is important for building muscle, but there are so many more benefits besides getting stronger. Researchers state that "exercise plays a crucial role in mental well-being, reducing symptoms of depression, anxiety, and cognitive decline. It promotes neurotransmitter release (serotonin, dopamine), enhancing mood, sleep quality, and psychological resilience" (Aliberti & Capunzo, 2025).

How much exercise might be good for us each week? The World Health Organization (WHO) recommendation is 150–300 minutes per week of moderate-intensity aerobic exercise or 75–150 min of vigorous-intensity activity, with higher duration and intensity enhancing cardiovascular and metabolic effects.

Exercise may be good for our skin as well! "Regular physical activity induces the release of myokines, signaling proteins that enhance collagen synthesis and skin elasticity" (Haykal et al., 2025).

Frailty and Longevity

Maybe the most important benefit of exercise is its powerful effect on reducing frailty. If you're an unpaid family caregiver or have a friend who is a caregiver, you have seen firsthand the negative impact that frailty can have on someone's ability to live an independent life.

Frailty is often the reason some older people don't 'bounce back' from illness or injury and take much longer to heal. Researchers share that frailty is the difference between one person recovering quickly from a stressor while another person with less functional ability and resilience never really returned to their previous level of activity (Candore et al., 2024). We all know of someone who was just 'never the same' after a major illness or accident. When we talk about healthspan, we need to talk about frailty. According to research, frailty is "associated with an increased risk of mortality, loss of activities in a normal daily routine, hospitalisation, physical limitations, falls and fractures" (Bruyère et al., 2017).

Frailty may end our healthspan, so it's important to implement positive lifestyle habits. Frailty is partly associated with several things we cannot easily control, including our age, being female, our ethnic group, and our education and income. The good news is that frailty may also be affected by things we can control, including cardiovascular diseases, number of chronic diseases and medical conditions we have, our functional incapacity, poor self-rated health, depressive symptoms, cognitive function, body mass index, and smoking and alcohol use (Bruyère et al., 2017).

The Clinical Frailty Scale evaluates an individual's frailty from 1 (Very Fit) to 9 (Terminally Ill). Stage 3 is the last stage before frailty appears, and people at stage 3 are categorized as not regularly active beyond walking. The scale really recognizes regular physical activity as the difference between being fit and needing help with activities of daily living.

Researchers utilized the UK Biobank to see if the Life's Simple 7 (LS7) could predict future frailty. They also looked at whether social isolation and loneliness also has an effect on future frailty. The research showed that "both a better midlife LS7 score and good psychosocial health status were associated with a lower risk of frailty over a 10-year follow-up period" (Wang et al., 2023).

American Heart Association (AHA) Life's Simple 7 (LS7) includes:

- Not smoking
- Healthy weight
- Healthy eating
- Physical activity
- Blood Pressure
- Cholesterol
- Blood Sugar

(Wang et al., 2023).

Psychosocial environment factors including social isolation and loneliness may also have an effect on healthspan and frailty. Researchers found that "social isolation and loneliness in midlife both increased the risk of physical, hospital, and comprehensive frailty." The researchers stated that these findings indicate that "frailty might be caused not only by physical problems, but also by psychological problems" (Wang et al., 2023).

Researchers also found that a six-month lifestyle intervention in frail adults resulted in changes to epigenetic aging and functional outcomes. Nutritional supplementation and an exercise program including progressive resistance training, cardiorespiratory, neuromotor and balance exercises, and stretching may delay biological aging and disability progression (Olaso-Gonzalez et al., 2026).

VO2 Max

VO2 Max is a measurement of cardiorespiratory fitness and a predictor of longevity. Research has shown that "physical fitness may influence disease risk and biological aging" and "a higher level of physical fitness slows down the speed of aging" (Nasser et al., 2026).

The easiest way to get a general idea of your current VO2 Max score is to either run for twelve minutes or 1.5 miles and enter the distance or time from the run into an online calculator to see your fitness level.

An alternative for those who aren't used to exercise is the Rockport 1 mile walk test. This test uses heart rate and time spent walking to calculate VO2 Max.

12 minute run calculator: https://exrx.net/Calculators/MinuteRun

1.5 mile run formula is: VO2 max = (483 / time in minutes) + 3.5

1 mile walk calculator: https://exrx.net/Calculators/Rockport

Conclusion

After I recovered from my facelift and found myself approaching menopause, I became interested in feeling as good as I looked. My overall goal transformed to focus on lengthening my health span and reducing the amount of time I would spend struggling with disease and disability before I die. I remembered hearing about "Blue Zones," and I wanted to learn about why some communities have a high percentage of healthy older people. What's their secret? How could I add some of these practices to my life?

I wanted to improve my health from the inside out and from smallest (my cells) to largest (my community). I added some easy self-care habits to my routine that can help support the telomeres and mitochondria in my cells while reducing systemic inflammation and oxidative stress throughout my body. I also wanted to add stress reduction practices to my day, improve my digestion, and find an exercise routine that I enjoyed which would preserve my strength and stamina. Looking outside my own body, I wanted to build a community of friends and loved ones I can both support and rely upon.

We started our conversation off by looking at some of the reasons people may get facial plastic surgery and shared some tips for recovery. Then we looked into the science behind improving health, including the difference between healthspan and lifespan; Blue Zones; the importance of mitochondria, telomeres, and digestion; the negative effects of inflammation and oxidative stress on aging, and the positive effects of stress reduction, community, and physical activity on longevity.

We learned about stress reduction tools, including:

- Diaphragmatic breathing / 5/5 breathing
- Cyclic Sighing
- Gratitude Journaling
- Heartfulness Meditation
- OM/AUM chanting and thirumoolar pranayamam (TMP)
- Progressive Muscle Relaxation
- Self-soothing touch
- Volunteering
- Yoga and other mind-body practices
- Yoga nidra

We learned about several ways to evaluate longevity, including:

- American Heart Association (AHA) Life's Simple 7 (LS7)
- Clinical Frailty Scale
- Longevity Preparedness Index (LPI)
- Optimal Cardiometabolic Health
- PhenoAge
- Short Physical Performance Battery (SPPB)
- Sleep, physical activity, and nutrition (SPAN)
- VO2 Max score

Knowing how healthy you are isn't difficult or expensive. The PhenoAge test estimates biological age. The Optimal Cardiometabolic Health; Sleep, Physical Activity, and Nutrition (SPAN) and VO2 Max tests focus on cardiovascular health. The Clinical Frailty Scale, American Heart Association (AHA) Life's Simple 7 (LS7), and Short Physical Performance Battery (SPPB) estimate risk of frailty and future disability.

The Longevity Preparedness Index (LPI) gives you insight on your overall preparation for a long, healthy life. It's relatively easy to get answers from these tests and use them to track how implementing healthy behaviors changes their results over time.

I hope that this guide has given you the information you need to successfully heal from your facial plastic surgery as well as the inspiration to focus on your health to ensure that your body feels as young as the face looking back at you in the mirror.

Resources

Aliberti, S. M., & Capunzo, M. (2025). The Power of Environment: A Comprehensive Review of the Exposome's Role in Healthy Aging, Longevity, and Preventive Medicine—Lessons from Blue Zones and Cilento. Nutrients, 17(4), 722 Open Access CC by 4.0

Balasubramanian, S., Janech, M. G., & Warren, G. W. (2015). Alterations in Salivary Proteome following Single Twenty-Minute Session of Yogic Breathing. Evidence-Based Complementary and Alternative Medicine, 2015(1), 376029. Open Access CC by 4.0

Balban, M.Y., Neri, E., Kogon, M.M., Weed, L., Nouriani, B., Jo, B., Holl, G., Zeitzer, J.M., Spiegel, D. and Huberman, A.D. (2023). Brief structured respiration practices enhance mood and reduce physiological arousal. Cell Reports Medicine, 4(1).

Boccardi, V. (2025). From telomeres and senescence to integrated longevity medicine: redefining the path to extended healthspan. Biogerontology, 26(3), 107.

Boon, J. T., Maxwell, C. A., & Layne, D. M. (2025, September). Caring While Moving: Case Studies on Physical Activity and Dementia Caregiver Well-Being. In Healthcare (Vol. 13, No. 17, p. 2205). MDPI. Open Access CC by 4.0

Boyd, C. J., & Ceradini, D. J. (2025). Current Trends in Facelift and Necklift Procedures. Journal of Clinical Medicine, 14(12), 4273. Retrieved from: https://www.mdpi.com/2077-0383/14/12/4273. Open Access CC by 4.0

Bozick R., Donofry S., Rancaño K. (2025, Aug. 6) New Weight Loss Drugs. https://www.rand.org/pubs/research_reports/RRA4153-1.html

Bravo, F. G. (2022). Neck contouring and rejuvenation in male patients through dual-plane reduction neck lift. Clinics in Plastic Surgery, 49(2), 257-273.

Brown, S. M., Humphrey, S., Marçon, C. R., Benvenuto-Andrade, C., Lipko-Godlewska, S., de Almeida, A. T., & Montes, J. R. (2025, November). Perceptions About Aging and Aesthetics: A Global Study of Adults Aged 50 to 80 Years. In Aesthetic Surgery Journal Open Forum (p. ojaf127). Oxford University Press. Open Access CC by 4.0

Bruyère, O., Buckinx, F., Beaudart, C., Reginster, J.Y., Bauer, J., Cederholm, T., Cherubini, A., Cooper, C., Cruz-Jentoft, A.J., Landi, F. and Maggi, S. (2017). How clinical practitioners assess frailty in their daily practice: an international survey. Aging clinical and experimental research, 29(5), 905-912. Open Access CC by

Candore, G., Accardi, G., Aiello, A., Baggio, G., Bellini, T., Calabrese, V., Carreca, A.P., Carreca, I., Masucci, A., Cattaneo, M. and Dato, S. (2024). Sex and gender in ageing and longevity: Highlights from an international course. Translational Medicine@ UniSa, 26(1), 15. https://pmc.ncbi.nlm.nih.gov/articles/PMC10980291/pdf/tmed-26-01-015.pdf. Open Access CC by 2.5

Caregiving for Family and Friends - a Public Health Issue. (2018). Retrieved from: https://www.cdc.gov/healthy-aging-data/media/pdfs/caregiver-brief-508.pdf

Chavda, V. P., Feehan, J., & Apostolopoulos, V. (2024). Inflammation: the cause of all diseases. Cells, 13(22), 1906. Open Access CC by 4.0

Deledda, A., Giordano, E., Velluzzi, F., Flore, G., Franceschelli, S., Speranza, L., & Ripari, P. (2022). Mitochondrial aging and senolytic natural products with protective potential. International Journal of Molecular Sciences, 23(24), 16219. Open Access CC by 4.0

Diez, G. G., Anitua, E., Castellanos, N., Vázquez, C., Galindo-Villardón, P., & Alkhraisat, M. H. (2022). The effect of mindfulness on the inflammatory, psychological and biomechanical domains of adult patients with low back pain: A randomized controlled clinical trial. PloS one, 17(11), e0276734. Open Access CC by 4.0

Dreisoerner, A., Junker, N. M., Schlotz, W., Heimrich, J., Bloemeke, S., Ditzen, B., & van Dick, R. (2021). Self-soothing touch and being hugged reduce cortisol responses to stress: A randomized controlled trial on stress, physical touch, and social identity. Comprehensive Psychoneuroendocrinology, 8, 100091.

Dziewiecka H., Buttar H. S., Kasperska A., Ostapiuk–Karolczuk J., Domagalska M., Cichoń J., et al. (2022). Physical activity induced alterations of gut microbiota in humans: a systematic review. BMC Sports Sci. Med. Rehabil. 14, 122. 10.1186/s13102-022-00513-2 Open Access CC by 4.0

Everly, G. S., & Ramirez, J. (2025). Longevity-Focused Wellness: Toward a Revolution in Workplace Wellness–

Slowing Down the Aging Process and Extending Healthspan for High Risk Groups and Public Health. Crisis, Stress, and Human Resilience: An International Journal, 7(2).

Faria, M., Ganz, A., Galkin, F., Zhavoronkov, A., & Snyder, M. (2024). Psychogenic aging: a novel prospect to integrate psychobiological hallmarks of aging. Translational Psychiatry, 14(1), 226. Open Access CC by 4.0

Flament, F., Maudet, A., & Bayer-Vanmoen, M. (2023). The objective and subjective impact of a daily self-massage on visible signs of stress on the skin and emotional well-being. International Journal of Cosmetic Science, 45(6), 761-768.

Garmany, A., & Terzic, A. (2024). Global healthspan-lifespan gaps among 183 World Health Organization member states. JAMA network open, 7(12), e2450241-e2450241. Open Access CC by 4.0

Gill, T. M., Murphy, T. E., Barry, L. C., & Allore, H. G. (2009). Risk factors for disability subtypes in older persons. Journal of the American Geriatrics Society, 57(10), 1850-1855.

Giridharan, S. (2024). Yoga and Telomeres: A Path to Cellular Longevity?. Cureus, 16(11). Open Access CC by 4.0

Giridharan, S. (2024a). Yoga Nidra: a promising complementary therapy for enhancing cancer care. Cureus, 16(9). Open Access CC by 4.0

Guo, X., Wang, J., Guo, Q., Zheng, K., Ni, B., Fan, X., & Nie, Q. (2026). HbA1c as an Independent Predictor of Peripheral Artery Disease: Nonlinear Threshold and Causal Evidence from NHANES and Mendelian Randomization. *Clinical and Applied Thrombosis/Hemostasis*, *32*, 10760296261437047.

Guralnik, J. M., Ferrucci, L., Simonsick, E. M., Salive, M. E., & Wallace, R. B. (1995). Lower-extremity function in persons over the age of 70 years as a predictor of subsequent disability. New England Journal of Medicine, 332(9), 556-562.

Haykal, D., Flament, F., Shadev, M., Mora, P., Puyat, C., Dréno, B., Zheng, Q., Cartier, H., Gold, M. and Cohen, S. (2025). Advances in Longevity: The Intersection of Regenerative Medicine and Cosmetic Dermatology. Journal of Cosmetic Dermatology, 24(7), e70356. Open Access CC by 3.0

Haykal, D., Flament, F., Suwanchinda, A., Zheng, Q., Rowland-Payne, C., & Colonna, A. (2025b). Predictive Biomarkers: A New Frontier in Bespoke Aesthetic Dermatology. In Aesthetic Surgery Journal Open Forum (p. ojaf155). Oxford University Press. Open Access CC by 4.0

Jeong, I., Cho, E.J., Yook, J.S., Choi, Y., Park, D.H., Kang, J.H., Lee, S.H., Seo, D.Y., Jung, S.J. and Kwak, H.B. (2024). Mitochondrial adaptations in aging skeletal muscle: implications for resistance exercise training to treat sarcopenia. Life, 14(8), 962. Open Access CC by 4.0

Jung, K. H., Yang, E. J., & Lee, W. (2024). Unilateral Platysma Muscle Rupture as an Effect of Using a Hard Wooden Block for Facial Massage. Archives of Plastic Surgery, 51(01), 027-029. Open Access CC by 4.0

Kloni, M., Heraclides, A., Panteli, T., Klonis, A., Rentzias, P., & Karagiannis, C. (2026). Incentive Spirometer in COVID-19: A Systematic Review. Journal of Clinical Medicine, 15(4), 1425. Open Access CC by 4.0

Koemel NA, Biswas RK, Simpson SJ, Rezende LF, Wang T, Bauman A, Raubenheimer D, Allman-Farinelli M, Cistulli PA, Ahmadi MN, Stamatakis E. (2026). Combined variations in sleep, physical activity, and nutrition and the risk of major adverse cardiovascular events. European Journal of Preventive Cardiology, zwag141. Open Access CC by 4.0

Kreouzi, M., Theodorakis, N., & Constantinou, C. (2024). Lessons learned from blue zones, lifestyle medicine pillars and beyond: an update on the contributions of behavior and genetics to wellbeing and longevity. American Journal of Lifestyle Medicine, 18(6), 750-765. Open Access CC by 4.0

Ladanyi, S., Adams, J., & Sibbritt, D. (2025). The Prevalence of Massage Therapy Utilization for Musculoskeletal Conditions: A Systematic Review. International Journal of Therapeutic Massage & Bodywork, 18(2), 5.

Lee, Y. C., Lu, C. T., Cheng, W. N., & Li, H. Y. (2022, September). The impact of mouth-taping in mouth-breathers with mild obstructive sleep apnea: a preliminary study. In Healthcare (Vol. 10, No. 9, p. 1755). MDPI. Open Access CC by 4.0

Levine ME, Lu AT, Quach A, Chen BH, Assimes TL, Bandinelli S, Hou L, Baccarelli AA, Stewart JD, Li Y, Whitsel EA, Wilson JG, Reiner AP, Aviv A, Lohman K, Liu Y, Ferrucci L, Horvath S. (2018). An epigenetic biomarker of aging for lifespan and healthspan. Aging (Albany NY), 10(4), 573. Open Access CC by 3.0

Li, S., Stampfer, M. J., Williams, D. R., & VanderWeele, T. J. (2016). Association of religious service attendance with mortality among women. JAMA internal medicine, 176(6), 777-785.

Li, R., Zhang, T., Cheng, Z., Yao, C., Meng, X., & Ma, T. (2025). Advancements of physical exercise and intestinal microbiota and their potential mechanisms. Frontiers in Microbiology, 16, 1595118. Open Access CC by 4.0

Malphrus, E. L., Perelmuter, S., Rubin, R., & Percec, I. (2024). Menopause in plastic surgery patients: an underrecognized and undertreated comorbidity. Plastic and Reconstructive Surgery, 154(4), 901-908.

Marxen, T., Shauly, O., Goel, P., Tsan, T., Faria, R., & Gould, D. J. (2023). The utility of lymphatic massage in cosmetic procedures. In Aesthetic Surgery Journal Open Forum (Vol. 5, p. ojad023). US: Oxford University Press. Open Access CC by 4.0

Mind and Body Practices (2025) Retrieved from: https://www.nccih.nih.gov/health/mind-and-body-practices

Morel, S. B., Macias, L. H., Chopra, R., Vorstenbosch, J., & Safran, T. (2025). Aesthetic submandibular gland resection: a review of complication incidence and prevention. Aesthetic Surgery Journal, 45(9), 869-874. Open Access CC by 4.0

Moszeik, E. N., Rohleder, N., & Renner, K. H. (2025). The Effects of an Online Yoga Nidra Meditation on Subjective Well-Being and Diurnal Salivary Cortisol: A Randomised Controlled Trial. Stress and Health, 41(3), e70049. Open Access CC by 3.0

Narenthiran, P., Smith, I. G., & Williams, F. M. (2025). Does the addition of manual therapy to exercise therapy improve pain and disability outcomes in chronic low back pain: a systematic review. Journal of bodywork and movement therapies, 42, 146-152.

Nasser, S., Keringer, J., Gu, Y., Boldogh, I., Ba, X., Higuchi, M., Kerepesi C, & Radak, Z. (2026). Physical Fitness Is Negatively Associated With DNA Methylation-Based Risk of Aging-Related Diseases. Aging cell, 25(4), e70467. Open Access CC by 4.0

Nichol, B., Wilson, R., Rodrigues, A., & Haighton, C. (2024). Exploring the Effects of Volunteering on the Social, Mental, and Physical Health and Well-being of Volunteers: An Umbrella Review. *Voluntas: international journal of voluntary and nonprofit organizations*, *35*(1), 97-128. Open Access CC by 4.0

Noordam, R., Gunn, D. A., Tomlin, C. C., Maier, A. B., Mooijaart, S. P., Slagboom, P. E., Westendorp, R.G., De Craen, A.J., Van Heemst, D. & Leiden Longevity Study Group. (2013). High serum glucose levels are associated with a higher perceived age. Age, 35(1), 189-195.

Nowakowska W, Grodzicka J, Winkowska A, Kłak I, Szerocki J, Bartnik K, Mazur K, Karalus M, Curyło W, Grudina A. (2025). The effect of lymphatic massage and physical activity on delaying signs of skin aging: A literature review. Open Access CC by 4.0

Okuda, I., Takeda, M., Taira, M., Kobayashi, T., Inomata, K., & Yoshioka, N. (2022). Objective analysis of the effectiveness of facial massage using breakthrough computed tomographic technology: A preliminary pilot study. Skin Research and Technology, 28(3), 472-479. Open Access CC by 4.0

Olaso-Gonzalez G, Millan-Domingo F, Garcia-Fernandez L, Garcia-Tercero E, Cebrian M, Garcia-Dominguez C, Carbonell JA, Casabo-Valles G, Garcia-Gimenez JL, Tamayo-Torres E, Gambini J, Tarazona-Santabalbina FJ, Vina J, Gomez-Cabrera MC. (2026). A Multidomain Lifestyle Intervention Is Associated With Improved Functional Trajectories and Favorable Changes in Epigenetic Aging Markers in Frail Older Adults: A Randomized Controlled Trial. Aging Cell, 25(2), e70376. Open Access CC by 4.0

Ornish D, Lin J, Chan JM, Epel E, Kemp C, Weidner G, Marlin R, Frenda SJ, Magbanua MJM, Daubenmier J, Estay I, Hills NK, Chainani-Wu N, Carroll PR, Blackburn EH. (2013). Effect of comprehensive lifestyle changes on telomerase activity and telomere length in men with biopsy-proven low-risk prostate cancer: 5-year follow-up of a descriptive pilot study. The lancet oncology, 14(11), 1112-1120.

Parsa, K. M., Gao, W., Lally, J., Davison, S. P., & Reilly, M. J. (2019). Evaluation of personality perception in men before and after facial cosmetic surgery. JAMA facial plastic surgery, 21(5), 369-374.

Patil, Y., Sabbu, K., Iyer, R.B., Philip, S.T., Nadhar, A.A., Thakur, K.S., Kadu, P., Thakur, M., Patil Sr, Y. and Iyer, R. (2024). Effect of Heartfulness Meditation on Oxidative Stress and Mindfulness in Healthy Participants. Cureus, 16(6). Open Access CC by 4.0

Picard M, Prather AA, Puterman E, Cuillerier A, Coccia M, Aschbacher K, Burelle Y, Epel ES. (2018). A mitochondrial health index sensitive to mood and caregiving stress. Biological psychiatry, 84(1), 9-17.

Pickart L & Margolina A. (2018). Regenerative and Protective Actions of the GHK-Cu Peptide in the Light of the New Gene Data. Int J Mol Sci. 2018 Jul 7;19(7):1987. doi: 10.3390/ijms19071987. PMID: 29986520; PMCID: PMC6073405.Open Access CC by 4.0

Poljsak, B. (2011). Strategies for reducing or preventing the generation of oxidative stress. Oxidative medicine and cellular longevity, 2011(1), 194586. Open Access CC by 3.0

Pujos, M., Chamayou-Robert, C., Parat, M., Bonnet, M., Couret, S., Robiolo, A., & Doucet, O. (2025). Impact of chronic moderate psychological stress on skin aging: exploratory clinical study and cellular functioning. Journal of Cosmetic Dermatology, 24(1), e16634. Open access CC by 4.0

Rabah, S.M., Alkhars, H.F., AlAlwan, A.Q., Albalawi, T.A., Alazzmi, H.A., AlQahtani, M., Alkhars, A.F., Rabah, S., Alkhars, H. and AlAlwan, A. (2025). Beauty Standards and Societal Influences on Facelift Surgery Decisions in Saudi Arabia. Cureus, 17(3). Open Access CC by 4.0

Reilly, M. J., Tomsic, J. A., Fernandez, S. J., & Davison, S. P. (2015). Effect of facial rejuvenation surgery on perceived attractiveness, femininity, and personality. JAMA Facial Plastic Surgery, 17(3), 202-207.

Reynolds, B., McDevitt, A., Kelly, J., Mintken, P., & Clewley, D. (2025). Manual physical therapy for neck disorders: an umbrella review. Journal of Manual & Manipulative Therapy, 33(1), 18–35. https://doi.org/10.1080/10669817.2024.2425788

Rieder, E. A., & Fried, R. G. (2021). Essential Psychiatry for the Aesthetic practitioner. Wiley Blackwell.

Rodriguez, C. I., Isobe, K., & Martiny, J. B. (2024). Short-term dietary fiber interventions produce consistent gut microbiome responses across studies. Msystems, 9(6), e00133-24. Open Access CC by 4.0

Salehi, B., Azzini, E., Zucca, P., Maria Varoni, E., V. Anil Kumar, N., Dini, L., Panzarini, E., Rajkovic, J., Valere Tsouh Fokou, P., Peluso, I. and Prakash Mishra, A. (2020). Plant-derived bioactives and oxidative stress-related disorders: a key trend towards healthy aging and longevity promotion. Applied Sciences, 10(3), 947. Open Access CC by

Sasada, M., & Guest, P. (2016). The facelift bible: Including the facelift diaries. Clinispa Limited.

Schwartz, N., Chalasani, M. L. S., Li, T. M., Feng, Z., Shipman, W. D., & Lu, T. T. (2019). Lymphatic function in autoimmune diseases. Frontiers in immunology, 10, 519. Open Access CC by 4.0

Smith, A. P., Sutherland, D., & Hewlett, P. (2015). An investigation of the acute effects of oligofructose-enriched inulin on subjective wellbeing, mood and cognitive performance. Nutrients, 7(11), 8887-8896. Open Access CC by 4.0

Taş, S. (2020). The effects of vibration and pressure treatments in the early postoperative period of rhinoplasty. Aesthetic Surgery Journal, 40(6), 605-616.

Teut, M., Brinkhaus, B., Stöckigt, B., Binting, S., Elies, M. K., Zwingmann, C., & Jeserich, F. (2025). Religion, spirituality, well-being and praying the Rosary: Results of a cross-sectional study from Germany. Journal of religion and health, 64(2), 1195-1221. Open Access CC by 4.0

Turska-Kawa, A., & Pilch, I. (2025). Psychopolitical and Psychosocial Predictors of Self-Perceptions of Aging Among Young-Old and Old-Old Adults. SAGE Open, 15(3), 21582440251374413. Open Access CC by 4.0

Twal, W. O., Wahlquist, A. E., & Balasubramanian, S. (2016). Yogic breathing when compared to attention control reduces the levels of pro-inflammatory biomarkers in saliva: a pilot randomized controlled trial. BMC complementary and alternative medicine, 16(1), 294. Open Access CC by 4.0

Wang Q, Zhou C, Dong C, Zhang J, Xie Z, Sun H, Fu C, Hao W, Zhu D. (2023). Midlife life's simple 7, psychosocial health, and physical frailty, hospital frailty, and comprehensive frailty 10 years later. Nutrients, 15(10), 2412. Open Access CC by 4.0

Wang, B., Szücs, A., Sandalova, E., Lim, Z.M., Horberg, E.J., O'Keefe, P.A., Island, L., Rosenthal, S. and Maier, A.B. (2025). Public views towards lifespan, healthspan, and Healthy Longevity Medicine in Singapore: a qualitative study from the HEalthy LOngevity (HELO) initiatives. Gerontology. Open Access CC by 4.0

Wang, Q., Wang, Z., Mizuguchi, K., & Takao, T. (2025a). Biological age prediction using a DNN model based on pathways of steroidogenesis. Science Advances, 11(11), eadt2624. Open Access CC by 4.0

Wang, R., Yin, X., Chen, Y., Wang, X., Shi, M., & Zhang, Y. (2026). Loneliness, social isolation, and biological aging: Evidence from two large population-based cohort studies. Journal of Affective Disorders, 121690.

Yegorov, Y. E., Poznyak, A. V., Nikiforov, N. G., Sobenin, I. A., & Orekhov, A. N. (2020). The link between chronic stress and accelerated aging. Biomedicines, 8(7), 198. Open Access CC by 4.0

Yeruva, N., Rodriguez, L., Romero, M., Aryal, A., Pina, L. A., & Saygi, M. (2026). Multifaceted benefits of xylitol in oral health: from caries prevention to periodontal therapy. *Bioinformation*, 22(1), 588.

Yuan, H., Shi, J., Gu, C., Yuan, J., Huang, C., Li, X., Zhou, K. and Qi, J.. (2026). Akkermansia muciniphila: A next-generation gut probiotic supporting neurorepair and functional recovery.

Neural regeneration research, 10-4103. Open Access CC by 4.0

Wang, R., Huang, X., Wang, Y., & Akbari, M. (2022). Non-pharmacologic approaches in preoperative anxiety, a comprehensive review. *Frontiers in public health*, *10*, 854673.

Witkowski, M., Nemet, I., Li, X.S., Wilcox, J., Ferrell, M., Alamri, H., Gupta, N., Wang, Z., Tang, W.H.W. and Hazen, S.L. (2024). Xylitol is prothrombotic and associated with cardiovascular risk. *European heart journal*, *45*(27), 2439-2452.

www.ingramcontent.com/pod-product-compliance
Lightning Source LLC
LaVergne TN
LVHW040516210926
848480LV00005BA/1479
9798996335206